THE CLINICAL I

❈ ❈ ❈

Scenes from a Doctor's Life and Practice

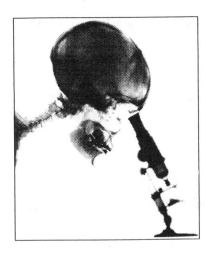

Irwin Siegel, M.D.

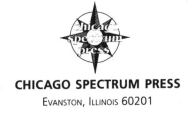

CHICAGO SPECTRUM PRESS

Evanston, Illinois 60201

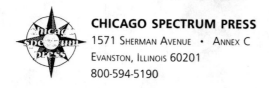

CHICAGO SPECTRUM PRESS
1571 Sherman Avenue • Annex C
Evanston, Illinois 60201
800-594-5190

Printed in the U.S.A.

10 9 8 7 6 5 4 3 2 1

ISBN: 1-886094-21-7

All of this
is for Joe.

"Non ridere,
None lugere,
Neque detestere,
Sed intelligere...."

"Not to lament,
Not to laugh,
Not to curse,
Only to understand...."
                    -Spinoza

ACKNOWLEDGMENTS

❊❊❊

No book is written alone. The author wishes to gratefully acknowledge the contribution of the following: Ms. Alice Thanner, for unparalleled secretarial support; Mrs. Jackie Abern, for expert typing; Ms. Cecile Wege, for first-rate transcription; Ms. Patricia Casey, for patient proofreading; Dorothy Kavka, CEO of Chicago Spectrum Press, for her skillful shepherding of the book through the critical processes of publication. Finally, I wish to thank all dramatis personae, patients and professionals alike, real and imagined, who continue to enlighten and entertain my clinical eye, never failing to engage *THE CLINICAL I.*

–Irwin M. Siegel
Evanston, Illinois
March, 1995

CONTENTS

❧ ❧ ❧

PREFACE

The practice of medicine is seldom as portrayed on television or in the movies. You can't adequately diagnose and treat a major clinical problem in sixty minutes with time out for four commercials. Medical practice is much more dramatic than the media would have us believe. In truth, its only similarities to show biz are that you are judged only as good as your last operation, and the show, no matter what, must go on.

Medicine is, at best, a mixed bag. It provides the excitement of challenging cases, the tedium of routine examinations, the joy of providing health and sometimes even saving lives, the suffering of illness and the sadness of death. It inspires the courage to make life and death decisions and, at the same time and to the same degree, the concern that you may be wrong. It frees you and it traps you. It offers temptations, makes demands more stringent, and pays rewards more beautiful and meaningful than those of any other life work I know. It quickly discovers and exploits weaknesses. It is funny, it is bewildering. It stretches from laughter to sorrow. It brings both pleasure and pain, and it is often difficult at any one time to tell with which of these you are dealing. It demands strength, but mostly it asks for humility. It evokes feelings I have come to understand but am not yet able to explain.

Everything written here is true. All of it happened. Some happened to me, some to him, some to us. But, it all happened. And it is these happenings, this human interplay, this work, this never-ending attempt to discover and own every part of ourselves which milks meaning out of the sometimes madness of life. It is this examination which finally brings the world into focus.

I am a doctor. Here are scenes from my life and practice. Here is the Clinical I.

DOCTORS

How do you describe what it is to be a doctor? The question is an existential one; a true doctor is what he is always becoming — is that why they call it practice? The profession of medicine is structured around a paradox. Physicians, like priests, which indeed they once were, constantly work to put themselves out of the business of doctoring. The young doctor is untested, thus unlimited. He is eager to prove his newly acquired skills. But he soon must recall the lessons of freshman physiology, remembering that inspiration is an active maneuver, expiration a passive one, and it takes both to breathe. In the work of medicine, the not doing is often as important (even more important?) than what is done. If you can err by commission or omission, you can also correct by either. During the magical process of healing, the heart works as well as the mind — why indeed separate them at all? And the heart works at rest as well as in motion; it simply couldn't contract without first relaxing. The trick is to know when to let well enough alone. The patient will tell you his diagnosis if you will but listen. The body will often heal itself, if only you don't get in the way.

There is one thing more difficult than describing what it is to be a doctor. That is being what a doctor should be.

What He Remembered Most

What he remembered most was the rough-woolen smell of his jacket and the fresh-washed coolness of his hands as they gently examined him. He also remembered the deference his parents paid him when he came to visit, taking his overcoat at the door, offering him a clean towel and answering his questions concerning the illness, quickly, quietly and with respect. All this in spite of the fact that he was an old family friend with whom his father had attended high school. This was his first and most meaningful contact with a doctor, and he felt that he, too, wanted to enter sickrooms, be treated with deference and heal with cool hands.

Much later, he visited his office which was located above a drugstore on South Ashland Boulevard. It was straight out of a Norman Rockwell illustration, the waiting room furnished in brown wicker, potted plants, and old, dog-eared *National Geographic*s. His consultation room even had a rolltop desk in glorious disarray strewn with medical texts, old prescription pads, and innumerable papers, torn-out articles and notes.

Later still (he was a junior in high school by then and President of the Zoology Club) he took him to the Michael Reese Hospital and let him witness an operation. He was fascinated by what he saw and sensed, and he vowed then to become a surgeon or perish in the effort.

He thought of all these things as he examined him, aged, severely diabetic, badly arthritic, almost totally blind. He couldn't do much for him, but he prescribed some pain medication and explained a way he could more comfortably transfer from his bed to the chair in which he sat for most of the day, where his wife read to him from medical journals, the prose and poetry of his life.

"It was nice of you to visit," she said as she saw him to the door, "especially considering how busy you must be. We hear such wonderful things about you, and Alex is proud that he played even a small part in starting you out on your career."

Leaving, he thought how he had begun to come full circle. It seemed as if all too suddenly he was physician to his doctor, parent to his mother and father. It was a strange feeling for he had not yet had time enough to make a full adjustment to the change of roles. Indeed, the child had died. And yet, the child still lived.

It Was Difficult to Believe

It was difficult to believe he was once a young man. But he had been, brown-haired and slim, interested and interesting. His was a middle-class general practice, and he did his job well. He knew how to triage the variety of medical and surgical problems which he attended in large number. He was competent to treat what he had to treat, yet also knew when to refer.

Then he started seeing nursing home patients. Slowly but surely he began to visibly age. His hair began to gray and thin and his abdomen to protrude. His shoulders became stooped and he hardly ever smiled. He took it all to heart. He always empathized and often sympathized with his increasing burden of feeble, toothless, rheumy-eyed, bed-wetting, sheet-picking, clientele. He was in constant battle with the hospital utilization committee and even the nursing staff.

"But who will take care of them if I don't?" he would exclaim in a tone of resignation, looking more tired than ever, even at breakfast.

And, indeed, who would? Still, he was the target for everyone's outrageous slings and arrows.

"What business does he have filling our valuable beds with such crocks?"

"I have trouble getting a chest pain or a GI work-up in, while he takes beds for patients who require nothing but feeding and diaper changes!"

And he keeps getting older. He even shuffles some as he makes his rounds. He has so identified with the senile objects of his ministrations that he has begun, in middle age, to look like a caricature of their agedness.

Yet wearing his infirmity like a threadbare secondhand coat, so obvious to all but him, he cannot diagnose, much more care for, himself.

Which of us, however, looks well after that particular patient?

▨

A Few Simple Things

He once read that a doctor travelling through the mountain villages of Nepal had been approached by natives with hideous deformities and incurable diseases. They wanted to be touched by the white doctor from the West. Apparently they believed that this simple laying on of hands would effect a magical cure.

"How long have you had pain?"

"It's been at least several weeks, and it's getting worse."

"My examination, confirmed by the x-rays we've just taken, reveals rather severely advanced degenerative arthritis."

"Is that a serious condition?"

"It's not life-threatening, but it's slowly progressive and it may get quite uncomfortable from time to time, particularly with physical or emotional fatigue or abrupt changes in the weather."

"You're right, those things do aggravate the pain."

"There's really not much to be done, except to reassure you that you don't have a more serious condition, such as an infection, tumor, or crippling inflammatory arthritis."

"That's a relief!"

"There are a few simple things you can do to minimize the frequency and severity of your pain. You must keep your weight down, use moist heat locally, take aspirin on a regular basis, and get plenty of rest."

"I do all those things already."

"So, there's not much else to be done."

"But you've done a great deal already, Doctor. Just having someone to talk to, who has enough interest to take the time to listen, has helped me immeasurably. And somehow I feel better since you examined me. It's almost as if your touching me was treatment in itself."

Before the Wounded

He met her in Jerusalem. Her name was Orlee.

"That means light, doesn't it?"

"'Or' means light. 'Orlee' means my light, the light that comes from me."

"That's a risky name to carry around during a blackout."

"You're teasing!"

"I guess so, but you see, my Hebrew name is Yitzhak, and you know what that means."

"To laugh."

"So, I'm just exercising my birthright when I joke."

"You speak very well Hebrew for an American."

"Not well at all. I studied some for my Bar Mitzvah. But it wasn't until I came to Israel that I learned my name. I wish my Hebrew was as good as your English, Orlee. Where did you study?"

"In school, and I listen to the news in English every day on the BBC radio."

"Well, you listen well, Orlee, and I don't say that lightly. Tell me, do you like being a nurse?"

"Yes, I like it, except when there is war."

"The work here at Hadassah must be very hard for the nurses, especially now."

"Yes, very hard, but still I'm sorry to leave."

"Leave? Where are you going?"

"Tomorrow I go to Rafidim in the Sinai. There are many wounded there, and the nurses are very tired. My friends and I will replace them for a while, so they can come back for a rest. The war is going badly, isn't it, Yitzhak?"

"Yes it is, but we'll win. We can't afford not to."

"They say we have already over a thousand dead, three thousand wounded. When, I wonder, will it end?"

"Well, Orlee, it started on Yom Kippur. I hope we're through at least by Succoth."

"You're teasing again."

"I joke so I won't weep, Orlee; but seriously, it must end soon. We're running out of men, out of ammunition, and out of time.

"Are you married, Yitzhak?"

"Yes, I'm married."

"And do you have children?"

"Yes, I have children, two children."

"You left your family to come here to help us fight the war?"

"Yes, I left my family to come here and help you fight the war."

"Why?"

"Because I had no choice, Orlee."

"But we're Israelis, we are always the ones without choice. You, an American, you have every choice."

"Not all borders are geographical, Orlee. Besides, I also came for a very selfish reason."

"What reason?"

"I came to find what's missing."

"And what is missing?"

"I don't know yet, but I'll know when I find it. Are you married, Orlee?"

"I was married."

"Then you are no longer?"

"My husband was killed in the Six-Day War."

"I'm sorry."

"Thank you, Yitzhak."

"Even a Yitzhak can't joke about that, Orlee."

"It's all right. Sometimes the whole thing seems like a joke. Maybe that's all it is. God's big joke."

"Will you have dinner with me tonight, Orlee?"

"Thank you, Yitzhak. It would be very nice to eat something other than hospital food, especially on my last night in Jerusalem."

"My shift in surgery is over at ten. I'll meet you at the main gate at 10:15. If I have to work into the midnight shift, I'll send word."

"I'll be waiting."

No more casualties arrived that evening. They met as planned and hitchhiked into the darkened city. The only restaurant they could find open was the coffee shop in the King David Hotel. The normally busy cafe was almost empty. None of the usual crowd of tourists, business men, and visiting dignitaries, only a few soldiers with their also soldier dates sitting seriously over their food at tables scattered throughout the small room. They slipped into a corner booth and ordered sandwiches and coffee from the meager menu.

"What will you do after the war, Yitzhak?"

"Same thing I did before."

"Are you happy with your work? Do you enjoy being a surgeon?"

"I'm happy being a doctor, I don't always enjoy being a surgeon."

"What don't you enjoy about it?"

"You have to act like you know what you're doing even when sometimes you don't. You have to always be strong and in control even when you're full of self-doubt."

"Do you doubt yourself now?"

"I've never been so sure in my life."

19

"Can I have another coffee, Yitzhak?"

"By all means."

"What does that mean, 'by all means'?"

"It means yes, Orlee, it means very, very yes. Now tell me, what do you plan after the war?"

"I think to work and save my money. I'd like to travel. I've always wanted to visit the United States. I hear so much about it. I've seen many movies of America. What's it really like, Yitzhak?"

"It's a very beautiful place, Orlee. But sometimes it can be very cruel. We have lots of plastic, and slums of course, both poor and rich ones, but there are no wars there. At least none outside the immediate family."

"I don't understand."

"You will when you visit. Finish your coffee, Orlee, and let's go for a walk."

They strolled down King David Street toward the old city. Entering through Jaffa gate, they passed the Tower of David, and turning right, took Zion Road to the Wailing Wall. The ancient city was abandoned, row upon row of metal shutters, locked like a line of obscene mouths tightly shut. Other than the two of them, the only other visible inhabitants were Israeli soldiers standing guard every hundred yards or so. They stopped to share a few moments of talk with each.

The Wailing Wall, too, was without other visitors. They approached it like children, silently and in awe, finally touching the massive stones, heavy and cool in the moonlight.

"It's the custom to write a wish and put it in the cracks between the stones," Orlee whispered. "It is said that if you do this, your wish will come true."

He searched his pockets for a scrap of paper, and finding a crumpled duplicate of a blood transfusion requisition, tore it in half. Each then wrote a wish, but before adding them to the thousands of others already stuffed between the temple's ancient stones, they exchanged papers and silently read each other's request. Their eyes met with no astonishment, only understanding. Both had wished for the same thing, each writing one word only — 'Shalom', peace. He kissed her then, and as he held her, she turned away and began to cry.

"Why are you weeping, Orlee?"

"I weep because I cannot joke. Because I'm sad, because I'm happy. Because my name is not Yitzhak, but Orlee. And even through I can make light, I cannot laugh, remember?"

"It is after midnight, and you leave early tomorrow for the Sinai. Where will you spend the night, Orlee?"

Sensing fully the unasked question, she turned again to face him, and standing on tiptoes to reach his full height, she whispered, "Yes, oh yes, by all means yes."

They walked slowly from the Old City, down the narrow, winding cobblestone passageways. They held hands, but did not talk. The air was cool and their footsteps the only sound in the war-darkened place. Exiting through the Damascus Gate, they hitched a lorry to Mt. Herzl, and then after a brief wait, an ambulance returning from the city took them the rest of the way to the hospital. He fumbled with the key to his room, almost losing it in the dark. Once inside, after making certain the blackout shutters were tightly drawn, he lit the small table lamp.

"Orlee," he said, "will I see you again?"

"I think not, Yitzhak."

"You will be careful of yourself, won't you?"

"I will try."

They very slowly and very gently undressed each other. Then they turned out the light and held each other tightly and for a long time. Their coupling was urgent and tender as desperately they sought meaning through the life-cherishing gift they shared. They slept briefly, awakening in each other's arms. They showered together, laughing as they held each other under the cold spray. There were no towels, so they dried with the still warm sheets. Then they dressed and walked to the main gait, where they silently waited for Orlee's bus to arrive. She boarded quickly, but turned at the last moment, her dark eyes looking at him, yet through him, toward the Sinai.

"Yitzhak," she said, "'Shalom' is not only the word for peace, it has other meanings as well."

"What else does it mean, Orlee?"

"It means hello, it means good-bye, and in the Old Testament, 'Shalom' also means complete."

"Then Shalom, Orlee."

"Shalom, Yitzhak, by all means, Shalom."

The door to the bus closed between them. Then, in a cloud of exhaust and dust, it drove away, and suddenly she was gone.

He stood there feeling the mounting heat of the day on the back of his neck. He stared at the now-empty place where the bus had been. Then he slowly turned and started to walk back toward the hospital. He had not walked far when he heard it, the ever-increasing distant drone. Looking toward the south, he sighted it as it first appeared over the hills, and he could plainly hear the now-familiar keening of the helicopter rotor, cutting the air like a saw as it sped toward the hospital like a crazed insect. It was a large Sikorsky. It would be carrying wounded from the battle in the Sinai. It was too hot to fight during the day; the battles were always at night, the wounded delivered fresh the next morning. He knew it would be full of casualties, and he started to run. Many injured, many burned. He ran faster. And as he ran, what was missing quite suddenly fell into place. They needed him. Indeed, they needed him, but, for the very first time, he realized how much he needed them. In that instant his life became strangely complete. For he understood that everything, even this, carried its own special truth. In his need, he no longer had to choose, because there really was no choice. He was alone, yet through the aloneness, he somehow felt a joyous link with everything and everyone. He was running free now, for the first time running free, only one thought in his mind as he sped toward the receiving ward, "I must get there, I must get there before the wounded!"

◪

Details

A plastic bag filled with bottles of half-used pills. She spills them over his desk.·

"I take them all. Nothing helps."

They include three pain relievers, two muscle relaxants, sleeping pills, two tranquilizers, and a narcotic.

Details

"Dear Doctor: This is to inform you that we represent the above captioned in a lawsuit on injuries sustained in an accident occurring on such and such a date, at such and such a place, for which, she informed us, she is currently under your care. Would you kindly send us a full medical report of her condition, including your examination, laboratory workup, prognosis, and any other medical information related to injuries incurred in this accident."

Details

"Dear Doctor, your case, Ms. So and So in room such and such, has been reviewed by the Utilization Committee and found unjustified for further hospitalization. Medicare benefits will cease for this patient commencing 72 hours from the date of this notification. Yours sincerely."

Details

"What kind of arthritis do I have?"

"The garden variety degenerative kind. It's not inflammatory or crippling."

"I thought last time you said it was bursitis."

"You have that, too. Bursitis is a cousin of arthritis."

"Didn't I once have tendinitis?"

"Yes. And you also had myositis, spondylitis, capsulitis, fibrositis and fasciitis!"

"You're confusing me!"

"Then don't ask so many questions. Just take your medicine."

Details

The incision should be six inches long and should begin one handsbreadth distal to the posterior inferior iliac spine, sweeping gently down the lateral aspect of the thigh. The subcutaneous tissue and fascia should be incised in line with the skin incision ...

The Senses

The smell of soap, of ether, of antiseptic as it is painted onto a patient's body. The smell of steamed instruments in a tray fresh from the autoclave, a moist hot smell. The smell of the inside of a fresh paper surgical mask, a dry smell, a cool smell. The obscene stinks of an autopsy. The smell of blood, dried blood, wet blood, a sticky smell. The smell of muscle as it is cut, of bone as it is tooled. The smell of sterile dressings, bandages, rollers, a white smell, a clean smell.

The slap sting in the palm of a well-passed instrument. The stiffness of fresh operating garb as you stretch the starch to push your arms or legs through a blouse or pants. The stretch and snap of latex surgical gloves. So thin and right, they are like a second skin. The Swiss-watch-tuned balance of an otoscope in the hand. Wet plaster, creaming as you mold it and warming as it hardens. Skin, soft baby skin, milky girl skin, tough man skin, wrinkled old skin, freckled skin, white skin, black skin, hairy skin, smooth skin, skin, skin, skin ... The sliding, grating, giving-up feeling of a broken bone as it yields to your touch and is once again straight.

The taste of sweat as it leaks into your dry mouth during the third hour of a tough case. The taste of hot, sweet coffee leisurely sipped in the surgeon's lounge between operations. The spicy taste of Italian food ordered in from the open-all-night local diner after a late emergency case.

The high-pitched rhythmic beat of the cardiac monitor. The deep breathing sounds of a patient anesthetized. The efficient swish of starched nurses' skirts. Oxygen bubbling through water at six liters a minute. The staccato cry of your on-call beeper. Ah, the senses, all the senses.

We Are All Accessories

We are all accessories to the crimes we commit. *"They asked me not to exert any heroic efforts to save him."* Remember, one should always prolong living, but never prolong dying *"I don't know the answers, but I do know that there are answers"*. The relatives visit, but what they talk about is not what they really think. *"Just rest comfortably, and eat everything on your tray, and you'll be well in no time at all."* The private nurse fluffs up the pillows, gives a back rub, sorts the mail and wonders about her next case. *"I hope it's as easy as this one; medicals are better than surgicals, not as many tubes to watch."* The intern makes his efficient rounds. *"How did you sleep last night? When was your last BM?"* The resident tests his clinical skills. *"Very interesting, his liver is down three fingers. Must have metastasis. We'd better run a liver profile."* The patient is a "good" patient, noncomplaining, permitting all, no questions asked. *"Just do your best, and have faith."* The scenario unfolds. Each in his appointed role. Yet, the final act is never entirely final. Such feelings, like a phantom limb, remain long after the wound is healed. Their half-life is forever. Omission or commission, we are all accessories to the crimes we commit.

❖

Physician Heal Thyself

"**A**re you enjoying the conference?"

"Immensely."

"I am too, but I don't know if I'd operate on as many fractures as they advise. And their instrumentation is very heavy."

"You're right, you have to be quite a mechanic to practice orthopedics these days."

"Did you get a chance to see the exhibits?"

"Not yet, I have a difficult time getting around in crowds."

It was only then I noticed the cane lying on the floor underneath his chair.

"An orthopedic surgeon with an orthopedic problem? I guess you're just another case of 'physician health thyself'."

"I wish I could, but I've got multiple sclerosis."

"I'm sorry to hear that."

"So was I when I was diagnosed five years ago. It started with a little weakness in my fingers, and then some numbness in my legs. I gradually got weaker until I had to sit during surgery and finally couldn't even operate that way. But, I'm fortunate. It hasn't affected my vision or my balance. I can get around using a single stick and I can still drive."

"So you limit your practice to the office?"

"Yes, my associates have been very understanding. I do mostly office orthopedics, diagnosis, simple manipulations and casts, injections, that sort of thing. I also do insurance examinations and disability evaluations. I'm the only one in town who can see a patient for a lawyer or insurance company without a three to six week wait for an appointment. I insist on taking my turn on emergency room call, but if anything big comes in, I have to call for help."

"Is your MS pretty well stabilized?"

"Oh, I notice a little progression in the weakness now and then, but I'm much better in the cold weather. I've been to all the specialists, Boston, New York, England, every place there is. I know as much about the disease as anyone else. There's no cure, you know. They don't even know what causes it."

"Well I hope you enjoy the rest of the meeting. Can I assist you in any way? Can I help you into the lecture hall?"

"Thanks much, but I prefer to make it on my own. It's been nice chatting with you."

As I briskly stepped into the crowd heading toward the conference hall for the afternoon session, the corner of my eye caught him in the effortful act of rising to his feet, using mostly his arms. He retrieved his cane, and after waiting until most of the crowd had disappeared into the hall, he started slowly to limp toward the lecture room. Then it occurred to me that I had forgotten to ask him why he was attending a conference on new techniques in the surgical management of complicated fractures. On second thought, I was glad I didn't. And anyway, the answer was obvious.

What Happened to You?

It's humiliating and you mentally replay the accident over and over again. It hurts and you limp. The x-ray is negative for fracture. The ankle begins to swell. You tape it. You hate to use a cane. How come no one ever told you that when you use a cane your arm aches after a while. You're the doctor, but suddenly you're addressed like a patient, and you don't like the role. And just how do you handle all those not-so-funny jokes everybody is making about "physician heal thyself." You sit still for a while and the pain goes away. Suddenly you shift your weight and it's back again, reminding you of your invalid state. And "invalid" is the right term to apply. The myth of your invulnerability is totally invalidated. You're reminded first-hand what it's like to need repair. Are all patients with a game leg as frustrated and angry at having to conserve energy, planning even the simplest act to minimize the need to walk? Why are the stairs suddenly so formidable (it's up with the good, down with the bad foot first, as you recall). And how long have we had all those dangerous throw rugs in the house? You realize that a leg is not only a very necessary piece of anatomy, but also a part of a body image and life-style. You wish people wouldn't stare, and you'd like to wear a sign saying, "Please don't ask me what happened." You feel silly, stupid, angry with yourself. And besides that, it hurts every time you step on it. It's a good lesson in humility, and no doubt, on balance, the patient empathy gained is well worth it, but still ...

Indeed, "What happened to you?"

Emergency Room Scene

Are we going to keep that attempted suicide or transfer it out? Don't know, we're still waiting for word from Cook County Psychiatric. It depends on whether they have beds or not. By the way, have they moved that DOA out of Booth 4? I've got to close this scalp laceration. I'll check it for you, but we've got what looks like an MI in the hall and I'd like to have the medical people go over him before you get settled in. O.K., triage is the magic word. Tell them they're lined up out the door and it's only 10 P.M. Looks like a long night ahead. Shall we call in the reserves? Only if they outflank us. That seldom happens; after all, it's easy to tell the good guys from the bad, we wear the white suits. I think we ought to see the bum with the GI upset next. Why? Because I think it's more than just a GI upset. His last vomitus looked like coffee grounds and, besides, he's been puking on the gentleman with the sprained thumb from the suburbs who couldn't get ahold of his private doctor this morning. How about the baby with the 104° fever? No signs of meningitis, and the nurse is alcohol-sponging him now. I hear there's a rumble in the park and the squadrols are on the way over. *C'est la vie,* what's another skull fracture among friends. Listen, I'd rather see the backwash from a dozen rumbles, tire chains and all, than one stab or bullet wound of the chest or abdomen. Those always come in three's and we've already filled our quota twice this week. I've got to find a place to work, what's in Booth 6? A couple of smoke inhalers from the fire. They're still taking oxygen. They'll probably have to be admitted. Are you finished with your coffee? Just. Then what do you say we go save some lives? Suits me, I haven't anything better to do at the moment.

Cafeteria Scene

Sam, come over here and sit with us, but bring another cup of coffee. You want one too, Burt? Make it two, Sam. As I was saying, I sure wish I could get out of this racket. I'm so damned rushed. And it's not getting any better. Somewhere in this rat race there must be me, and I sure would like to say hello now and then. Don't complain, you GP's have it made. You ought to try surgery for awhile. In addition to tying your kishkes into knots, now we have to worry about whether the patient is going to sue us because she doesn't like the looks of her hemorrhoidectomy scar. And what's worse, she often wins. Sued has the same letters as used, but that's the price you pay for wanting to play God. Why don't you guys complain about problems we can do something about? There will always be work even though we're one of the few professions constantly trying to put ourselves out of business. There will always be patients, and anyone who doesn't have a hernia yet, just isn't carrying his share of the load. Now the food here at Mount Sinus Hospital is something else. I think we ought to bring the matter up at the next general meeting of the medical staff. Freud said there are only two great tragedies in life: One is not getting your heart's desire; the other is getting it. Spoken like a true shrink, but I suppose that depends upon what your heart's desire is. Looking at another specialty from a disgruntled point of view toward your own is sort of like looking at another man's wife on Saturday night. You forget that she also appears in a housecoat and curlers on Monday morning. Sit down, John. Hey, where did you get the chop suey? They didn't have it out when I went through the line. You've got to know the chef. He owes me a favor. I took care of his girlfriend last week. I hope it wasn't for typhoid. No, nothing like that; just a lump in the breast, but it wasn't the Big C. Ah cancer, my favorite disease! You are a fiend, even though you do the best liver biopsy in the hospital. Speaking of livers, how is Bill getting along? I understand his latest profile shows his past has finally caught up with him. It's not his past so much, it's that self-treatment all these years. Remember what old man Christenson used to say, "A doctor who treats himself has a fool for a doctor and a damned fool for a patient!" Al, did you get a chance to see that patient on Four Northwest? You mean the one with the knee pain? Yes, what did you think? I think it's an IDK. What's that? An Internal Derangement of the Knee. It doesn't sound like anything too specific? Are you sure it doesn't mean "I don't know"? A little bit of that, too. In any case, we're going to have to look in the joint and see what we can put back together for him. Well, that's enough caffeine for the morning. I've got to make rounds. See you guys later. How about you? Why not. See you at lunch. Yeah, see you at lunch.

WOUNDS

An emotional wound is like a physical wound. It needs time and care to heal. Unlike physical injury, however, mental suffering leaves a scar which is often larger than the wound it fills.

To treat such wounds, to avoid such scarring, the physician must tune his brain, his heart and his hands to the same wave length. The product of such accord is more effective in healing than the penetrating frequency of a laser beam.

In the final analysis, there is no such thing as an uninteresting case. There is only the uninterested doctor. The challenge is to change like a chameleon on a checkerboard to accommodate the particular needs of each patient, that is, if you're interested. The core problem is that you can't always cure. But, you can always care. And, if you are patient with yourself (and your patient), you come to see that all of nature's forces finally add up to zero; otherwise, nothing would work, ever.

Waiting is difficult, even if you know what's going to happen, as you often do. It gets lonesome, but you're never really alone. There's always you and, if you're interested, there's you watching you. But this means expanding your consciousness, owning every part of yourself. It means trusting and touching. It's not easy. No one ever said it was.

❄

He Sat in the Wheelchair

He was so steeped in the machismo of his Spanish origin, that it was painful for him to even mention the matter privately to a doctor.

"I can't be a man anymore," he whispered, averting his eyes, "I can't perform my husbandly duties anymore."

I tried to sound convincing. "You realize, of course, Mr. Lopez, that that's not all there is to being a husband, or even a man."

"But, Doctor, you don't understand. I used to be so strong, so capable. I used to dance, to run, always the first, always the best."

"I can't promise you'll run or dance again, Mr. Lopez, but if you're patient with yourself, and try not to get emotionally upset, and if your wife is understanding and accepting, there are ways."

He sat in the wheelchair with his wasted hands in his lap. His wavy hair was heavy and black, his dark moustache well manicured. He wore a silk robe and a paisley ascot to match. He looked like a Spanish duke casually receiving a guest. Except that in this case, the guest was uninvited. He suffered from amyotrophic lateral sclerosis, and not only would he not be able to dance or run again, but within a few years he would develop difficulty swallowing, and then breathing, and then he would die. He was looking at me now, and the burning in his dark eyes told me that he also knew all of this. It was difficult to turn away from his searching, questioning, pleading look, and my neck began to ache from the effort of not avoiding his gaze.

Please Mrs. Greenberg

"It's all over, Mrs. Greenberg, you're back in your own room now."

"But ... where are the others, where have they gone?"

"What others, Mrs. Greenberg? There are no others, only you. The operation is over, your hip is fixed, and you're back in your own bed. We'll get you up soon and in a day or two you'll be walking again."

"The rest of the barracks, where have they gone?"

"What barracks, Mrs. Greenberg? This is no barracks. This is a hospital."

"They've taken them all to the chimneys! I am the only one left now! Why didn't they take me, too? What did I do to be punished like this?"

"You're confused, Mrs. Greenberg. Don't you remember where you are?"

"They're all in flames by now. Mina's thin legs are burning, Rachael's old hands are burning, Sarah's beautiful red hair is burning."

"Please, Mrs. Greenberg, calm down now. You're temporarily confused. This sometimes happens with someone your age after an anesthetic. I'm going to give you an injection to calm you down. You'll be all right when you wake up. You'll be all right, just wait and see."

"They're all in smoke now, all in smoke, floating up to heaven. I'm the only one that's left. Just me alone. Why? What did I do to deserve this? Why me alone? Why me? Why?"

The Telephone

The telephone connects me to the world. Its secret dials and switches are another mouth and ears, its wires and cables extensions of my own nerves. In the beginning there was silence, and then Ma Bell created the telephone.

"Hello Irv, this is Aaron. I've got a problem. She's a 52 year-old female who had both breasts removed for cancer at Mayo's last year. She's got extensive pulmonary metastasis and is breathing on a third of one lung. She fell this morning and the x-ray shows a fracture through tumor in her right hip. What do you suggest I do?"

"Hello, dear. I just wanted to remind you to pick up some dog food on the way home tonight. And, oh yes, bring me a large can of those small peas you like. I've a beauty parlor appointment this afternoon, so I won't be home till late, and I'll have to throw together a tuna casserole for dinner. You don't mind, do you?"

"Irv, this is Eugene. Look man, you have to move some of those chronic backs in the house. The Utilization Committee is clamping down on all overstays. Under the new government regulations, hospitalization of most of these people will be cut off within the next 48 hours. I don't like it any more than you do, but there is nothing I can do about it. It's the law now, and we've simply got to cooperate with the government."

"Hello Doctor. I still have the pain. It never seems to go away. Can't you do something about it?"

"Good afternoon Doctor. This is Attorney Gross. Would it be convenient for you to give a deposition in the Stinewall case next Thursday at 1:00 in my office?"

"This is Mike in the emergency room, Doctor. You'd better come quick. We've got a suicide attempt and it's both wrists cut to the bone."

"Hello Dad. I just wanted to check what time you're getting home. I really could use the car tonight."

"This is the 5th floor nursing station, Doctor. Mr. Green, your patient in 502, insists on checking out of the hospital against medical advice. We can't restrain him. What should we do?"

"Good afternoon Doctor. We're taking a survey on the life insurance needs of physicians in the Chicago area."

"I can't thank you enough Doctor. You saved my life. I'll never forget you, and you'll always be in my prayers."

"You're the one who's responsible for all my pain and trouble. I regret the day I stepped into your office. The next one you'll be talking to will be my attorney."

The telephone, always the telephone. Who couldn't talk to me and who couldn't I talk to on the telephone. Maybe even God. If I could only remember the number.

Smoke

She was one of them.

The number tattooed on her forearm told me so.

Thin, pale, totally gray, 50 looking 70, and frightened to the point of terror.

"It pains. All over it pains. My shoulders, my back, my legs. Oh, how it pains."

Her uterus and ovaries were removed in a Nazi concentration camp when she was eighteen years old.

"Please help me, Doctor. It hurts so much. All the time. Everything hurts."

Her ugly abdominal scar was stretched and thin. Its whiteness matched the color of her hair. My fingers burned as I touched it.

"The pain is with me all the time. I can't get rid of it. I even wake up at night in the dark with the pain."

How could I explain that her scar was larger than the wound it filled. How could I tell her there was no cure for that kind of pain?

"If I could just get some relief, even temporary relief. If I could just sleep."

After all, it wasn't my fault. My hands are clean. I swear by Apollo, the physician, the Aesculapius and health and all heal, and all the Gods and Goddesses that, according to my ability and judgment, I am without guilt.

Yet, when will they stop appearing, these numbered ghosts? They escaped, but can we ever?

Before she left, I fled the room. It smelled of smoke.

Home

"He wants to marry me, Doctor, what do you think?"
"What to you think, Janice?"

"I don't know what to think. I just wonder why he wants to marry me."

"Because you're an attractive woman and, besides, you're gentle, understanding, kind, everything a man respects and desires."

"I just hope he's prepared."

"Prepared for what, Janice?"

"Why, prepared for me, what else?"

"He's the only one who can answer that. But why are you so disturbed that he wants to marry you?"

"Well, in the first place, he's a handsome, strong, normal guy."

"And this disturbs you?"

"Only because I'm far from being a normal girl."

"Does he love you?"

"He says so."

"What does his family think?"

"They think he's crazy."

"And your family?"

"They think we're both crazy."

"Do you think you're crazy?"

"I don't know. I think I love him. I certainly need him. But I can't help wondering whether he really loves me or is just trying to prove himself to himself. I want to be loved, Doctor, not used."

"Nobody loves anybody the way everybody wants to be loved, Janice. Your doubt is healthy, but give yourself time. Think about it. Talk it over with him. And get some outside help if you feel the need. With real caring you can make a life, you can have a home together."

"A life, perhaps. But a home? When I see others walk, Doctor, it seems to me that this wheelchair is the only home I'll ever have."

You Bet Your Life And Limb

Groucho: Well, it's been nice talking to you. You're a lovely couple, and I'm sure you'll get married and live happily ever after right after the show. But now it's time to play "You Bet Your Life and Limb." You know the rules, and if you say the secret word, you win $100. It's a common word. Something everybody wants but seldom gets.

Announcer: *(off stage)* The secret word for tonight is "Cure," folks.

Groucho: All right, then, for your category you selected "Fatal Diseases." For each question you get sixty seconds to decide on a single answer between you. Remember, the more the question is worth, the harder it is. How much do you want to bet on your first question?

Female Contestant: $100, Groucho.

Groucho: All the way, huh! O.K., here's the question — "What is the five year survival rate for a 35-year-old woman, mother of two children, suburban housewife, active in school and community affairs, adored by her husband and friends, with advanced cancer of both breasts, and extensive metastasis to the lymph nodes of both axillae, after bilateral radical mastectomy, radiation and chemotherapy?" You have one minute to decide on an answer.

(Clock running on camera. Theme song playing gaily in background)

Groucho: O.K., your time is up. What answer have you decided on?

(Hurried whispering between couple — on camera)

Groucho: Please, no help from the audience.

Female Contestant: Less than ten percent!

Groucho: Correct! You're exactly right. Less than ten percent!

(Audience applause)

Announcer: You now have $100.

Groucho: Well, you did great with that question. You certainly must keep abreast *(cigar in mouth, leer toward audience)* with medical progress. *(canned laughter)* Let's see how well you do with the next question. How much will you bet?

Male Contestant: Ninety dollars, Groucho.

Groucho: Remember, you have one minute for one answer. Here's the question: A nine-year-old red-headed, vivacious, little girl, an only child, good student, excellent in sports, who takes ballet after school and plans a career in dance, develops acute leukemia. What is her life expectancy?"

(Clock running. Musical background. Camera pans in to intense concentration on faces of contestants)

Groucho: Your time is up. What's your answer?

Male Contestant: Do you mean life expectancy from the time of the diagnosis or after a year or two of intermittent hospitalization with multiple blood transfusions?

Groucho: I'll take either answer.

Male Contestant: Well, I'd say less than five years in either case.

Groucho: Absolutely right. You win $90.

(Audience applause)

Announcer: You now have answered two questions correctly and you have $190 between you. What will you bet on question three?

Female Contestant: Eighty dollars.

Groucho: Well, so far, you're doing fine. We've really been picking your brains and you're bleeding our bank dry *(winks at audience as he taps ash off cigar)*, but I'm sanguine about the outcome. So here's your third question. Now listen carefully. "A 12-year-old boy is the product of an uncomplicated pregnancy and birth. He is apparently normal until after four, at which time he begins to show signs of progressive weakness and disability. A diagnosis of muscular dystrophy is made. He gradually loses the ability to run, then walk, then stand. He is confined to a wheelchair at age 10. His extremities gradually weaken until he requires a motorized lift for transfer from wheelchair to toilet. He can no longer feed himself. His spine develops a severe curvature. However, his intelligence is normal and, all the while, he excels in any activity not requiring the use of his disabled extremities. What can be done to save his life?"

(Clock running. Background music)

Groucho: O.K., what answer have you decided upon? *(Frantic last minute consultation between contestants)*

Contestants: Nothing!

Groucho: These two are amazing. They've answered three in a row! You're absolutely right. Nothing can be done to save his life!

(Audience applause)

Announcer: Well, this is exciting. You've now answered three correctly. And you still have a chance to say the secret word and win $100.

Groucho: Well, I hope that last question didn't weaken you too much *(rolls eyeballs toward ceiling — audience laughter)*. Now here's your final question. What will you bet?

Male Contestant: seventy dollars, Groucho.

Groucho: All right, for $70, "A 40-year-old physician has spent 13 years acquiring an education in his specialty. He has an active practice, but also finds time for teaching and research. He's been married to a nurse since his sophomore year in medical school, and his wife worked to support his education until their first child was born. He's just beginning to pay off some of his outstanding debts and has been thinking about moving from his city apartment to a small home in a nearby suburb. One day during surgery, he begins to lose vision in both eyes. An extensive evaluation reveals an expanding intracerebral lesion. A craniotomy is performed and a diagnosis of malignant neoplasm is made. The tumor is so extensive, it cannot be removed surgically. Cobalt irradiation as a palliative is described. What is his prognosis?"

(Clock running. Musical background. Contestants silently concentrating — on camera)

Groucho: All right, for $70, what is the prognosis?

Female Contestant: We think it's poor, Groucho. In fact, it's so poor, we think it's negative.

Groucho: You're absolutely right. You win $70. His prognosis is zilch.

(Audience applause)

Groucho: Well, you sure got ahead with that one *(on camera — broad grin)* and you answered all four questions correctly. Your total winnings are $340. Tell me now, how come you two know so much about fatal diseases?

Female Contestant: *(Somewhat embarrassed, averting eyes and grinning slyly)* Well, Groucho, I myself had breast cancer. In fact, your first patient just about describes me.

Male Contestant: I guess I'll have to admit that I knew the answer to the second question because I have a child with leukemia.

Groucho: I thought there was something fishy going on. But how did you know the answers to the last two questions?

Female Contestant: It was just a lucky guess, Groucho. We figured that because the topic was "Fatal Diseases," all the conditions mentioned would be incurable.

Groucho: Clever, clever! Well, you didn't say the secret word, but you split $340 between you, and it doesn't matter anyway because the secret word was "cure." And you guessed it, there is no cure. So we don't pay off on that one. Anyway, you're both good sports, and I'm sure you'll make lovely music to-gether, a beautiful malady, that is *(puffs on cigar — audience laughter)*. So good luck to both of you, and thanks again for playing "You Bet Your Life and Limb."

While We Await the Wounded

Nervously,
we stand, huddled in the dark,
under a tense
Jerusalem sky,
counting each
his own life's hopes
while we await the wounded.

Silent,
the ordered fluids hang
ready
the stacks of dressings lay
how many?
how severe?
We whisper
while we await the wounded.

Suddenly,
the helicopter's grating
clawing at my heart,
for soon the stretchers,
warm with blood,
the smell of burned skin,
screaming,
the taste of pain.

Why are the nurses sleeping in corners?
Why are the instruments so warm to touch?
Why are the starts so quiet,
so indifferent?

While we await the wounded.

Jerusalem, October 1973

How Do You Feel?

"How do you feel?"
"Not any better, perhaps worse."
"Did you follow my instructions?"
"I don't remember what you suggested."
"I told you not to lift. I told you it would strain your back."
"Well, I have to lift at my job."
"I told you to lift from the knees, but not from the back."
"I could try that."

"I advised you to use some heat, hot baths, hot showers, a heating pad."

"I thought I was coming down with the flu and didn't want to take a chance using heat. I thought I'd get a chill afterwards, so I didn't use any."

"Did you take the medicine I prescribed?"

"Most medicines upset my stomach. I figured this one would, too, so I didn't get the prescription filled."

"You could take it after meals or with an antacid."

"I suppose so."

"Have you been resting your back? Lying down on a firm surface? Did you get a bed board for your bed?"

"My husband doesn't like a firm bed. He says it bothers his back. I haven't gotten around to getting a bed board, but I guess I could."

"My record shows that I ordered a surgical garment for you. How does it fit?"

"I didn't buy it. I thought I'd better try wearing a girdle first to see if it helped."

"Well, did it help?"

"No, not a bit."

"So, how do you feel?"

"Not any better. In fact, no better at all. Isn't there anything you can do to make me feel better?"

You're The Doctor

"You're in perfect health."

"I want another opinion."

"All right, you're very ill."

"Good, I feel better already."

"I'm glad, anything else I can do for you?"

"Don't you think I need a shot?"

"Of course you do. What did you have in mind?"

"Penicillin."

"What dose?"

"You're asking me? You're the doctor!"

"That's right, I am. For a minute there you had me fooled."

❊

A Peculiar Confusion

A peculiar confusion sometimes occurs when I am signing out charts. I can't for the life of me remember what some of the patients look like. It seems in a way so ludicrous. The record room ambience, the whole signing out charts process. Going over all those pages of notes and orders. Looking again at the pulse and temperature record, reviewing the laboratory results. All without the patient there.

Name, address, phone number, occupation, Social Security number, date, marital status, insurance, age, birth date, sex, religious preference, next of kin, room, bed, hospital number, date of admission, etc., etc. The busy miscellany of data and control. Food for the hungry computer.

Primary admitting diagnosis, secondary diagnosis, complications, procedures, operations, condition on discharge — recovered, improved, unimproved, not treated, deceased (autopsy performed?).

Each folder, of course, represents a human drama, often a tragedy, sometimes a lucky break, occasionally a joy (normal obstetrics), always a crisis of sorts. Just look at those shelves bursting with lives. No pain here though, no screams, no bleeding from the pages, no cold, hard tubes in warm, soft openings, no needles, no knives, no stink, no fear.

"Hello there, Mr. X, aren't you uncomfortable lying on top of Mr. Y and under Mr. Z?"

Through the miracle of modern dictation, I have just confined Messrs. X, Y, and Z to the hospital archives, to rest in peace forever, or at least until they are microfilmed. They may be recalled by the Utilization or Patient Care committee, or even subpoenaed by some lawyer hot on the trail of personal injury or malpractice. But they are silent now, unresisting, uncomplaining, they do not elicit sympathy or concern. They no more challenge understanding or skill.

And yet, in some strange way, they impress me. For here in my right hand I hold two weeks of agony, followed by the death of a child, balanced on the left by a full-term cephalic delivery of a seven and one-half pound normal male. But do they really balance? Can they ever balance? Indeed, are they only symbols? And is that why they have no faces, at least none that I can at the moment remember?

Feelings

Not only do each of us have similar feelings, problems and needs, but on close scrutiny it would seem the lives we live are very alike. True, the length and locale may vary, the dimensions and quality may differ, but in a very real sense, externals aside, we are all brothers and sisters under the skin. On its own, the meaning of each life is much the same.

To see this, it is necessary to slice experience very thin, much as a microtome sections a surgical specimen so that microscopic examination can be made at the basic, cellular level. An event, like a tissue, must be dissected by the imagination beyond the obvious, to the level of its simplest elements, if we are to reach that authentic layer of experience where reality hides. It was a wise man, indeed, who once said, "Truth, like beauty, when unadorned, is adorned the most."

He Tried to Understand

It was best done when he was on an out-of-town professional visit because there was less chance of discovery and embarrassment in a place where he wasn't known.

It started innocently enough. Leaving his hotel to go to the meeting one morning, he stumbled and twisted his ankle. It was only a mild sprain, but he limped for a block or so. As he tried vainly to keep up with the morning downtown pedestrian traffic, he noticed people watching. This upset him. He wondered why. Suddenly he realized he had never been the object of this kind of observation. He limped on trying to understand his feelings. What was it like, really like, to be a patient and not a doctor? What if the limp were permanent? What if it were progressive? Was the attention always a discomfort, or were there comforts, too? He tried to understand.

Limps were his stock and trade. He knew the subtleties of each type and could mimic them perfectly. At different times, in different places, he would try on a different one for size. The dropfoot of the polio. The circumduction drag of the hemiplegic. The scissoring gait of the spastic. People would stare or very pointedly avoid looking. He tried to understand.

Why did he do this? What did it authenticate? Was it really out of a need to understand, or had he also been averting his eyes? Had he been looking through instead of at? He felt trapped inside his own head. Was this the guilt? The anxiety? The crippling worse than any limp? He tried to understand.

47

❈

It Wasn't Funny

It wasn't funny.

"He's just like his father was, never telling me what's really on his mind, always sneaking off someplace. Won't eat what I cook. Won't even change his underwear until I tell him he has to."

"Is there some specific complaint this visit?"

"Complaint? There's nothing but complaints! But you can't get anything out of him. You can't pin him down long enough to get him to complain. I'm the one who has to do the complaining, and I've plenty of complaints. Just look how skinny he is. Thin as a rail. And pale. Won't eat the good meals I prepare. Would rather stuff himself with hamburgers, french fries, soda pop, and doughnuts. Junk food! That's all it is. Junk food!"

I turned to my patient. "What have you got to say about this, Leslie? Let's hear from you."

"I dunno, I guess I just like what I like."

"Do you have pain anywhere? Have you been sleeping well?"

"He tosses and turns all night. Groans and moans. He must have pain some place."

"I dunno, I dunno." Leslie now averting his eyes and restlessly shifting from foot to foot. "She made me come here, I dunno."

"Somebody will just have to take him in hand, Doctor. Ever since his father passed away, he hasn't been the same. A boy needs a man around the house. Someone he can look up to. Not that his father was that kind of man. Weak, you know, unsteady, not reliable. Nonetheless, a boy needs someone to look up to. I've had to be both parents to him since his father died, but he's really getting out of hand now."

What to say, what to do? Who to talk to first? The bitter widow, or Leslie, her 36-year-old son?

It wasn't funny.

◪

Somebody's Going to Pay for This!

"**S**omebody's going to pay for this!"

She was a middle-aged woman, in no apparent physical pain, but affronted and angry.

"Where does it hurt?"

"Can you imagine it, a crack like that right there in the sidewalk at State and Madison, the busiest corner in the world, can you imagine it!"

"What did you injure when you tripped?"

"With all the graft just three blocks away at City Hall, you'd think they'd find a few dollars to repair the sidewalks!"

"Did you lose consciousness on falling?"

"When I think of all the taxes I've paid to this goddam city and how little I get back!"

"When did this happen, was it this morning or this afternoon?"

"I've already called my nephew who's a lawyer. He'll be in touch with you for a report."

"Just calm down a minute and tell me exactly what happened."

"I'll sue them for a million dollars."

"Just tell me where it hurts."

"Somebody's going to pay for this!"

◪

The Bully

He was the neighborhood bully. I remember when he mercilessly beat a smaller boy over a trivial misunderstanding.

It was an oppressively humid summer day, and all of us watched with fearful fascination as he bloodied his victim's face in the hot dust of the school playground. Terrorized by such brute force and unable to stand the sight any longer, we fled to the dark comfort of our separate homes, to mother and iced tea, to the cool solace of things familiar, but he didn't stop. He beat the boy unconscious.

Later, yet early even for one of his aggressive bent, he got very big with women. He made out and he used to brag of it.

"I tell them to powder the tits and perfume the box, and I'll be right over," he would say and we believed him.

He was incorrigible in school and, finally, his distraught mother sent him to a military academy in the vain hope that once and for all he would be disciplined.

He wasn't, and one day in a display of ridiculous bravado he attempted to outrace a streetcar to the local station, was struck, and lost a leg above the knee.

He was fifteen years old when this happened. I remember it well because afterwards I couldn't sleep for several nights. I kept awakening, feeling my own legs to be sure they were still there.

After that he disappeared from the neighborhood and also from my thoughts. Then came the war, and after the war the university, medical school and practice.

I next saw him fifteen years later, and a recognition of who my patient was came upon me slowly, as if I were blowing the dust off a book, forgotten and only now taken from its shelf and slowly opened to the pages of the past.

"I'm having trouble with my artificial leg, Doctor. It seems to be rubbing a sore on the back of the stump." He spoke softly and with obvious deference.

"Your name sounds familiar to me. Have I ever seen you before?" I asked.

"No, I don't believe so. I was attending a clinic on the south side, but I recently moved north and it's too far to travel to get medical help. I live in the neighborhood and I got your name from the hospital."

It was then that I realized who he was, but I let the matter drop. I attended to his leg, suggested some changes in the fit of the prosthesis and prescribed a salve for the irritation of the stump. I also recommended that he rest for awhile to let the sore heal.

"I can't do that, Doctor, this is my busy season and I have to hustle to make as much money as I can right now."

"What do you do for a living?" I was really curious.

"Well, I sell ribbons to florists, and in two weeks it will be Mother's Day, which means a lot of business for them and they'll need a lot of ribbons. So you see, I have to be on my feet."

Mother's Day ... ribbons ... artificial legs and ulcerated stumps ... "powder the tits and perfume the box" ... violence and blood on a hot afternoon in a dusty playground ...

I have since wondered why I didn't tell him who I was. Perhaps it's because I sometimes doubt I really know.

It's an Ego Trip

It's an ego trip.

You can become a pediatrician and be a giant in the land of midgets. Or you can become a neurosurgeon and tinker in the inside of somebody's head. If aggression is your problem, you can cut skin or break bones, and it's all socially acceptable. You can finger openings, peek down tubes, handle excreta, and nobody will blink an eye. In fact, they'll even pay you for it. Whatever your bent happens to be, it can be satisfied.

If it's men you like, you can be a urologist; if it's women you hate, you can go into OB-GYN. If you want to really play God and be held accountable to no one, you can become a psychiatrist.

It's an ego trip.

But you have to keep riding the horse even if you fall off, especially when you fall off.

The last time you did the operation it failed, miserably failed. You have to get back on the horse — you have to ride again.

The indications for the surgery may come up again, or they may not. But, you have to get back on the horse. You have to show that you can ride.

"The operation will help you. I think we can be pretty sure of a success." The last one failed, miserably failed.

Like I said, it's an ego trip.

◪

Named

Baby Boy Doe, 12 hours new. Five pounds plus of pink neo-natal plumpness. All survival reflexes in working order. The umbilical stump necrosing nicely under its clamp, and that awful, twisted foot hanging like a sick question mark from an otherwise normal leg.

It was such a pathetic foot. Hardly bigger than an adult thumb. Such a pitifully misshapen little foot. The physician's hand could easily enclose it.

Talipes (the foot) equino (pointing down like a horse) varus (curving as a sickle). Talipes equinovarus. Such a tiny club-foot.

Baby boy Doe, still nameless, up for adoption. Baby boy anonymous. Baby boy clubfoot — nameless — Doe.

He carefully examined the deformity. He would manipulate the foot and apply a plaster cast. He would repeat this every two weeks. Gradually the malformation would be corrected. Because the tissues were new and flexible, they would respond to the gentle urging of his hands. But it would take time, and he must not lose patience and push too hard else he irrepara-bly damage the tiny limb.

His hands would sculpt the foot. They would know just how much pressure to apply and where and for how long. And as he did this, his hands and the foot would somehow become as one. They would draw energy from the foot, and the foot would respond to their craft and straighten. Both then would grow in strength, and it would be difficult to separate them.

Baby — nobody's child. Soon a stranger will share his name with you. Until then, these hands will be your father. They need you as certainly as you benefit from their skill. For through you they are acknowledged and defined. In this very special way, both of us are named.

The Hospital

Everything he could ever require or desire was there. It was a microcosm of the world, self-contained and total in its experience. There was birth and death, happiness and sorrow, pain and pleasure, labor and rest, there was even love. It became his nuclear and his extended family, and he came to know its moods and secrets. There could not for long be rejection of feeling there. It would surface to tell soon enough. Though status was apparent and a pecking order adhered to, it was neither spiteful nor resented. As I said, a family, where you could get angry or be angered at, but you would not hurt, nor be harmed, and certainly never alienated.

What a love-hate feeling he had for the place. With what intricate poise his mind kept the thousands of sensations it daily fed him in balance. He liked it best at night. It was more his own. The three to 11 crew was always looser, and his footsteps in the quiet corridors brought back sweet and awful memories of moonlighting hospital jobs during his student days. It was both castle and workhouse to him, school, laboratory, factory, jail and home. The happiest two hours of his day were the hour he arrived and the hour he departed. Over the years it had assumed a character, a personality which he had adapted to, but, in part, was still testing. More than any woman it was mother, wife and daughter to him; more than any man, father, brother and son. As he made his rounds each day, he knew which wards had problems and which had none, which rooms held death and which held hope, knew which lab tech was engaged to a young medical student to be married after graduation that summer, and which aide was sleeping with which orderly. He also knew which doctor had had a recent heart attack and was patiently awaiting the second (and final?) one. He knew who had recently joined the expensive country club, whose daughter had just had a positive breast biopsy, whose son had just graduated law school, whose had just dropped out of high school, whose wife was now working in the office, and whose was suing for divorce. He knew who had taken on a new man, who had lost a partner and was now working twice as hard. He knew who was sending to whom, who didn't like whom, who was avoiding whom, who was loving whom. He knew, most of all, his own feelings of interest and concern, of discomfort and distress, of wonder and surprise.

And all of this he touched and added to himself.

Clinic Scene

They sit on the hard-wooden benches like passengers in a Greyhound Bus Station after midnight. Some awake, some asleep, each with his own thoughts. Some reading, some staring blankly into space, some whispering with their neighbors. A few even bring their lunch, realizing the wait will, as usual, be long. Occasionally, a child will run about the room — by himself, or chasing, or chased by another. A sick infant will stir and whimper a bit in troubled sleep until his mother soothes his half-conscious fear. They wait patiently (definition "Patient": to bear with composure.). Some wait for a cure, all for help, and a few for a bus that will never arrive.

He stood apart from the rest and his suit, although old and threadbare, was clean and well pressed. He wore a Hamburg and carried a cane. He had a well trimmed, gray moustache and what appeared to be expensive dental work.

"I lost it all in the Depression and I never made a recovery. Even so, I try not to feel sorry for myself. It hurts to accept charity. I don't feel like one of those on Welfare. Dignity is important to life. At least to mine. I never sit in the waiting room. I always stand to one side. I appreciate your taking the time to listen to all this, Doctor. I know it has nothing to do with my physical complaints, but it's important for me to have someone listen. You are the only doctor who's ever helped me on with my coat after a clinic visit. It's kind of you, Doctor. Very kind, indeed."

(Definition "Clinic": one patient and one kind doctor.)

He had a stroke. It left the right side of his body paralyzed. His mouth sagged on the right as he drooled for lack of facial muscle power. He wore a brace and used a cane. He also suffered motor aphasia. He couldn't put together a two-word sentence, but he could understand everything that was said to him. He was locked forever into himself, and medical science had nothing to offer him. Case closed.

"Do you specialize in this disease?" the wife asked eagerly.

"No, I'm not a neurologist. I'm just an intern," he replied, at once flattered and embarrassed by the question.

"Then maybe you can help him because his problems are internal, you know. They're inside his head."

Each was a book in itself, a play in itself, an essay, a song, a story. A world in itself. Though often caught in the impersonal reflexive, something kept growing inside him, moving with the laughter and the sorrow, demanding to be touched.

"I thought as long as I came along with him this time, you could take a quick look at my leg."

He had just spent twenty minutes with her husband. There were eighteen more patients waiting and he was an hour behind.

"You see, I've had this pain for at least the last six months. It comes and goes. I can't remember injuring the leg. There's been no swelling or other change. Just the pain."

Two for the price of one.

"Here, just have a look (off comes the shoe, down rolls the stocking), just a peek; it will only take a second."

Sometimes, life itself can be an altered state of consciousness.

"Soak it in hot water."

"I can't. There's no hot water in my apartment."

"Use a firm bed."

"I can't. I sleep on a couch."

"Come back in a week."

"I can't. I haven't the car fare."

"Give him the medicine very four hours."

"I can't. I have to leave him with his sister who is too young to trust."

"Rest."

"I can't. I have to work."

"Eat a well balanced diet."

"Ha, ha, ha."

"You're going to die."

"Ha, ha, ha, ha, ha ..."

"Why are you laughing?"

"Because I'm already dead."

An Italian proverb has it that illnesses tell us what we are.

"How old are you?"

His voice reverberated as if an echo chamber were inside his head.

"I'm 84 and I'm tired."

He worked as a waiter in the main dining room of a downtown hotel. He hustled.

"You're going to have to slow down now, Sam" (just as in an echo chamber). "I'll give you some medication for the pain in your hips and we'll get you a cane, too. But mostly, you're going to have to slow down now."

Medicine, as a wise man once said, should be practiced as a form of friendship.

There are always 18 or 80 or 180 waiting. There would always be patients waiting. That's what patients did. They waited, with or without composure.

"I wouldn't lie to you, we make a little cut here and we thread this wire through your vein, up your arm, into your heart."

"Does it hurt?"

"No, it doesn't hurt."

Or it does hurt. Or we make an incision here, or we inject something there. We listen and we advise and we prescribe and we touch and we cut and we sew, and that's what we do. And we succeed and we fail — and that's why they call it practice.

The benches are empty now. How polished they are from the innumerable backsides that for years have shifted there restlessly. The lights are off and the clinic is dark. It is quiet until tomorrow. Yet it is not entirely empty. One patient remains. He is always there. He is first in line and last in line. When the others are there, he is there. And when the others have left, he remains behind. He is of all and with each. He turns to you, and his eyes speak the same plea, ever so softly.

"Doctor, I'm sick. Please ... please, let me heal you."

An Empty Bed

One of the advantages of having an office in the hospital is that after hours you can visit cases admitted that day without having to make an extra stop on the way home.

In the middle of an especially busy afternoon, he was informed by the hospital office that his patient, Mrs. Tillie Rappaport, was to be admitted to bed 225. He could not, offhand, recall the patient, but this wasn't unusual as he managed

57

a large practice and frequently arranged for hospital admission weeks or even months in advance. He noted the name and room number and after he finished office hours, around six o'clock, he walked over to the second floor to seek out his patient.

He chatted briefly with the three to 11 nurse who accompanied him while he checked a post-op from the morning. It was a routine check, the patient was comfortable; so it only took a few minutes. Then he headed for bed 225.

It was just beginning to turn dusk as he entered the two-bed room. You know, the kind of early autumn evening when the light is heavy and everything, even indoors, looks a little vague. It's too luminous to turn the lights on yet, and yet it's almost dark enough to do so. It's just a perfect in-between time. Anyway, it was obvious that bed 225 was empty. So he turned to the patient occupying the other bed in the room, thinking a mistake had been made. He looked at her name plate to verify this idea and found he was wrong. Although difficult to read in the waning light, the name tag told him she was Frieda Seltzer, not Tillie Rappaport.

"You came to see me, Doctor?" Frieda inquired with anticipation.

"I'm sorry, Mrs. Seltzer, I didn't come to visit you," he replied.

Then wishing to verify that the other bed was, indeed, reserved for his patient, he stepped across the room and bent over the bed, trying to see if it had been tagged for the elusive Mrs. Rappaport. As he hovered over the bed squinting at the name tag (it was now dark enough to make reading a problem), he heard Mrs. Seltzer mutter to herself in amazement, "Oy vay! There's a mishuganah doctor in my room. He's come to visit an empty bed!"

N

Committees

The hospital is run by committees. There are over a dozen such. Most important is the Executive Committee. In close pursuit, however, are the Utilization Committee and the Patient Care Committee. There is also the Tissue Committee, Infection Committee, Therapeutic Committee, and so forth. In fact, the only thing that seems to be lacking is a committee on committees. But perhaps that's the function of the Executive Committee. Then there are the ad hoc, post hoc, and ergo propter hoc committees.

Most committees meet monthly. Have you any idea how many man-hours (high priced ones at that) this involves? I wince when I think how many operations, patient visits, hours in the research laboratory are taken up by the endless work of committees. The committees I have served on, and they have been many, take themselves very seriously. Important matters are discussed at interminable length. Every committee member is given the opportunity to speak, and speak each does. Committee meetings stimulate pontification rather than brevity. It's been said that a committee is a group of people who keep minutes and waste hours. The mere presence of a secretary taking such minutes seems to inspire the desire to speak, not only for eternity, but also everlastingly.

After everyone has spoken his piece, a vote on the matter is taken and the question usually referred to another committee. Just the other day, I spent a restless hour in the grip of the Infection Control Committee. The issue was whether or not a new antiseptic detergent for hand cleansing should be introduced into the hospital. I tried to point out that what was needed was not a new hand cleanser but an in-service education program to teach hospital personnel to frequently wash their hands. I remarked that we were putting the cart before the horse if we thought we could increase antisepsis through the use of a new cleansing agent when we didn't insist on the use of gloves and masks for all wound inspections and dressing changes. These heretical remarks earned me the chairmanship of a subcommittee for further study of the problem.

Not that committees are entirely useless. True enough, as one wag noted, "A camel is a horse designed by a committee," but then again, camels are sometimes useful, and perhaps Lindbergh's flight would have been even more sensational if it had been arranged by a committee.

Some say that God is dead. I happen to know he isn't. God is very much alive indeed. He is a committee.

After The Operation

"**A**fter the operation, how soon can I get back to swimming, doctor? Exercise is very important to me."

"You can swim as soon as the few stitches are out. In fact, it will help rehabilitate the knee."

It was to be a routine arthroscopic operation for removal of a torn knee cartilage, and I was pleased to be dealing with an active patient, eager to rehabilitate himself after surgery.

"How about jogging, handball, that sort of thing?"

"All in due time. Soft tissue healing usually takes a week or two and then you should wait until the joint is strong enough to withstand the strain of heavy use. We'll give you some special exercises both before and after surgery to make sure you get back into your athletic program as soon as possible."

"That sounds great, Doc. My internist gave me a head to toe checkup just last month, and he says I'm in perfect condition, so I guess I have nothing to worry about."

"Nothing at all, I'd say."

"Well, I'm happy to hear that. I wouldn't want to break my pace now. Since I moved into that Uptown swinging singles apartment complex, I really set a style for myself. They have great facilities. A pool, a sauna, all sorts of planned social events. By the way, I assume I can start to dance as soon as I begin to walk?"

"Just about. As long as you don't strain the knee until its ready."

"O.K. I'll watch it, but I like to keep up with all the new dances, particularly the fast ones, the ones that are a little wild."

"I leave that to your discretion. You're not a child, and I'm sure you'll use common sense. Just let your knee tell you what to do. If it says 'ouch!', it means it wants you to take it easy."

"O.K. Doc, I'll do what you advise and the knee says. But the operation won't hinder my sex life, will it?"

"Only during the period you're hospitalized, and some people have even managed to not let it interfere during that time."

"Well, that's great, just great. Sex is very important to me. You'd be surprised how many notes inviting me for coffee or dinner I get in my mailbox at the apartment. There are sure a lot of lonely women and lovely ones at that. I'd hate to lose or even temporarily lessen my manhood."

"There's no chance of that with this operation and, knowing you, little chance of anything else doing it. Probably not for the rest of your life."

"Well thanks, Doc. I'll see you next Wednesday. When did you say the admitting office would call me?"

"About 8 A.M. You'll check in shortly after noon. I'll see you then."

He was well built, lightly tanned, conservatively dressed, and had lost most of his hair. He was 75 years old, a widower with three married children, and I never cease to be amazed at the strength of the expression of the life force in some people. It almost matches its weakness in others.

SURGERY

Stripped to its basics, it really doesn't seem like so much. After all, it is only cutting and sewing. The first surgeons were barbers. Ever wonder about the red and white stripes on a barber pole? These represent the colors of blood and bandage. In fact, it took a long time before the barber/surgeon's guild was chartered. The Company or Guild of the Barbers of London received its charter from Edward IV in 1462. And a special charter for surgeons was created 13 years later. In some parts of the world, even today, it's only the practitioner of internal medicine and its subspecialities who carries the title "Doctor." Surgeons are still plain old "Mister." Let me assure you, though, surgery is very special, and so are surgeons, or at least they should be. In the first place, its best practice requires a kind of synesthesia, where most of the sense organs function as one, everything ultimately focusing through an exquisite muscle memory upon the hands, which are the surgeon's other eyes. It's also very much a thinking man's game: what you don't do once with your head, you'll have to do twice with those hands.

One doesn't surgerize with impunity. In a way it's a violation. Cutting into a human body was not reckoned in the original scheme of things. There are both indications and conditions for each operation. The indications make the procedure necessary, the conditions make it possible. The patient should both require the operation and be able to undergo it. Another important condition is the comfort of the surgeon. Uncomfortable surgeons either dawdle or hurry, and the thoughtless operator soon finds that the only defense the unconscious patient has against the inept surgeon is to bleed.

I suppose the most rewarding and, at the same time, the most fearful aspect of surgery is the responsibility. "Respondiat superior," as our legal brethren say, "The surgeon is responsible not only for his actions but for all those under his direct supervision." This, of course includes everyone from the scrub nurse to the orderly. For this reason, an operation is the only situation I know of where one good idea is worth more than two excellent ones. Ultimately, the surgeon is the only one responsible.

Surgery is indeed a tense situation. Threefold tense - present, past and future. The surgeon must at one and the same time be keenly aware of what he is doing, what he has just done and what he plans to do next.

Yes, all we do is cut and sew, but every time we do it, we go straight through the eye of the needle.

The Most Difficult Thing Of All

The most difficult thing of all is simply to keep going. To endure and carry on, in spite of failure, albeit afraid.

He changed into the loose-fitting operating garb quickly, not joining the early morning banter of the surgeon's dressing room. As always, the starched, pajama-like clothes felt crisp and efficient as he slipped his arms through the shirt and tightened the drawstring around his waist. The conductive canvas shoes fit his feet like comfortable socks. He locked his locker, slipped the keys into his back pocket, and stepped into the operating room corridor.

There was the usual bustle of accelerating preparation, so the eight o'clocks could be started on time. When he arrived at the scrub sink he nodded hello to several other surgeons who had already begun their wash. Then he meticulously cleaned his glasses with anti-fog solution, slipped on a tight paper cap, making sure all his hair was tucked underneath, and tied on a disposable mask. He noticed that the inside of the mask smelled like the inside of the cheap paper Halloween masks he used to buy at the Five and Dime. He tore the cellophane off a sterile scrub brush packet, adjusted a comfortable flow and temperature of water with the knee faucet and, noting the time on the overhead clock, began his ritual ten-minute scrub. First his right hand, the thumb, index, middle, ring and little finger; then the palm, the back of the hand, in a circular fashion, up the arm to the elbow. Finally, a rinse from the fingertips proximally. The left hand, in the same manner. Then begin with the right again.

He was concerned about the case. So worried in fact that it had kept him awake most of the night. Although he had successfully performed the procedure a number of times, he had really fouled up the last time, injuring the patient's sciatic nerve. The damage could have happened at one of several points during the operation, a long and exacting procedure. It was too early to tell whether it was temporary or permanent, but in either case, he was the one at fault. The incident had severely shaken his self-confidence and had occupied his thoughts since it happened the week before, pushing everything else aside. He felt as if his carefully programmed life was suddenly disordered; as if something was seriously out of place, preventing everything else from running smoothly. He had relived the operation dozens of times trying vainly, if not to rectify, at least to understand the situation. Perhaps he was just tired, perhaps his judgment was not as sharp as it should have been, perhaps, perhaps, perhaps. Ashamed as he was of making such a mistake, he had discussed the matter with several close colleagues.

"Don't worry, it's a reported complication," one said.

"Everyone makes mistakes; you're not perfect," said another.

"The only way to avoid complications is to stop operating. Besides, it's only a mistake if you make it twice," said a third.

Nonetheless, he felt depressed and wished he hadn't undertaken the last case and was nervous about the similar problem he was to face in a few minutes.

He noted that he had scrubbed an extra two minutes for good measure. He rinsed his hands for a final time, and holding them in front of him at shoulder level, walked toward the room assigned to him for the morning. "I wonder if this one will be as difficult, either during or after," he thought as he backed through the swinging door to avoid contaminating his hands. He turned around to see his patient already anesthetized on the table. He and the anesthesiologist simultaneously nodded in recognition of each other. He said hello to his resident and intern who were already gowned and gloved. He asked the nurse if several of his special instruments were sterile and in the room; she assured him they were. He studied for the last time the x-rays placed in the view box while he carefully dried his right arm from fingertips to elbow with one end of the sterile towel the nurse handed him, and then flipping the towel to its opposite end, he repeated the procedure on his left. Then he pushed his arms through the operating gown which the scrub nurse held toward him, allowing the circulating nurse to tie it behind at the neck and waist. He thrust his hands into the latex gloves which, stretching, fit like a second skin, put on a back gown and tied it in front, wiped the excess powder off the gloves with a damp sponge, and accepting a sterile towel from the scrub nurse, started to drape the patient.

He suddenly felt very alert, yet very calm.

A Word From Our Sponsor

"*Your patient has stopped breathing, Doctor. I'm afraid he's gone into cardiac arrest!*"

"*Quickly then, call a Code Blue and prepare the cardiac shock machine. In the meantime, I'll open the chest. Scalpel!*"

He crossed the room and sighed himself into bed. The sheets felt cool, and he found himself eagerly reaching for the friendship of sleep.

"I've got an early scrub tomorrow morning, dear. Can't you turn the TV off?"

"I can't right now. Dr. Gannon is just about to save another life. Why do you always ask me to turn off the set at the most exciting moment?"

He was so tired it almost didn't matter. His mind a kaleidoscope of slow motion scenes, like the old "flickers," his day residual moving slowly under the review of the strobe light of memory.

"*Knife, suture, clamp. Time?*"

"*Thirty seconds, Doctor. I think we may have a chance to save him!*"

The tensions of his surgery that morning. Three hours spent within millimeters of someone's spinal cord. The sweat-drenching, bone-aching exhaustion of it all.

"*I'm bag-breathing him, and his color is returning, but still no complex on the EKG monitor.*"

The late, rushed rounds. Having, like a chameleon, to change his personality and approach to meet each patient's special need.

"Is the defibrillator ready? O.K., turn on the juice!"

The gulped lunch accompanied by two table-side consultations.

"That's good, set it up a notch. Now, give him another shock!"

The consult with the family of a dying patient. The dash to the emergency room to treat the attempted suicide. The meeting with the Education Committee to discuss the house staff's lecture series.

"We're getting a tracing now. Is the rhythm normal? Good!"

His late afternoon office hours. The endless stream of patients. The wounds, the dressings, the swellings, the pain. The complaints, the queries, questioning, examining, treating, explaining. The phone calls, the scheduling, the interminable reports.

"His pulse is full, his rhythm is regular, and he's breathing on his own now, Doctor. I think we've saved him!"

His early evening hospital rounds on the way home, checking the post-ops. Having late coffee with the second shift, scheduling his morning surgery. Stopping for a quick review of the new library journals on the way out.

And the last thing he remembered just before completely surrendering to himself was how very much he loved it all. How, in spite of the hours, the fatigue, the never-ending concern, how in spite of always giving, and sometimes beyond the most, he could never see himself doing or being anything or anywhere else.

"Wasn't that exciting, John! They always manage to save patients in Hospital Center, even under the most trying circumstances. Well, don't you agree. Answer me, John. Why don't you answer me? Are you asleep already? I wonder what you're so tired from? I'm sure you never had to work as hard as Dr. Gannon."

And now, a word from our sponsor.

❊

Legacy

He had to hurry because Professor Warren was operating, and the small amphitheater would be filled to standing room only. He arrived half an hour early, but other students were already climbing the narrow staircase to the observation balcony. The date was October 16, 1846, the place the Massachusetts General Hospital, Boston, Massachusetts.

He turned toward the stairwell. It was slower than the elevator, but he liked to keep moving and be by himself just before surgery. It calmed him down, yet, at the same time, psyched him up for the tensions of a big case.

It was a long climb and he was out of breath when he reached the top. He was pleased, however, to find an empty seat in the first row. He quickly sat down on the narrow wooden bench and adjusted his arms on the metal railing to assure an unobstructed view of the operating pit below. He was too excited to join the murmur of casual student banter surrounding him. He enjoyed surgery. He wanted to be a surgeon. He felt there was a central truth here and he had to pay it due respect with attention and silence.

Silence. He didn't like to talk while operating, except, of course, to ask for instruments or point out some pathology or technique to the assisting resident or intern. Too much talk wet his mask and risked contamination of the wound. Besides, he didn't want his concentration disturbed, even by himself. He felt that the real skill was more in the head than in the fingers. That was the central truth of it.

Two nurses were filling metal basins with water and arranging instruments on a wooden table. Their starched skirts reached to the floor and rustled like wheat in the wind as they moved efficiently about the narrow room. It was now ten o'clock. The amphitheater was packed and all preparations for the operation made. A heavy door at the far end of the room was opened by a porter standing nearby and the patient was wheeled in.

The patient was wheeled in. He had been premedicated an hour before and now lay quietly on the metal cart. The scrub nurses had opened their packs and carefully lined up the instruments in ritualistic order on two OR tables and a Mayo stand. The room was diffused by a glareless, shadowless light, and the soft green color of the operating garb, sheets and drapes, blending with the cool blue of the floor and wall tiles, created the illusion of working somewhere underneath the sea. The anesthesiologist entered and began to calmly arrange his tubes, tanks, and valves.

The patient stirred. His frightened eyes scanned the amphitheater, searching for some relief from the tumor eating away at his jaw. The door opened a second time and Doctor John C. Warren, 69 years old, professor of surgery, one of the founders of Harvard Medical School, strode into the room in black cutaway and tie, his first footsteps echoing from the wooden floor as he crossed to his patient, an entourage of seven assistants and guests following closely behind. Four guards stood ready to hold the struggling and shrieking patient during the operation to follow. His agony should be brief. Warren was noted as a swift and skillful operator. He turned to his patient and wished him a good morning.

He turned to his patient. "Good morning," he said, "Dr. Glass here will be giving you your anesthesia. Don't worry about a thing. All you have to do is relax and the next thing you'll know, the operation will be over and you'll wake up in the recovery room." He had changed into operating garb, shoe covers, cap and mask, and now he stepped to the scrub sink for a careful ten-minute cleansing of his hands. He began to think. He was worried about the procedure. The tumor was deep. He would have to be extra careful in order to get it all.

The week before he had a visit from a young Boston dentist, William Morton, who was also a Harvard medical student.

He had been experimenting with the use of a chemical called ether to relieve pain in dental procedures and asked for an opportunity to give a demonstration of his method on a patient undergoing a surgical operation. With some ambivalence Warren consented. It was fruitless to hope that operations could ever be performed without pain, but if there were a chance, any chance at all, however small, it was worth taking to find out. He nervously waited for Morton to arrive, repeatedly checking the time on the watch he carried in his right hand vest pocket. After five minutes, he turned impatiently to the amphitheater, explained the delay, and finally said, "As Dr. Morton has not arrived, I presume he is otherwise engaged. Therefore, gentlemen, I think we had better begin."

Begin. When does one ever begin? After one ends, he thought. One seems to arrive only to depart and perhaps it's always a beginning of sorts, every day, even every minute. Halfway through the scrub he poked his head into the operating room. "Five minutes more to wash, Jim, then we begin, time to pass some gas."

"Gas, gentlemen, gas, nothing but more hot air. I am disappointed but not surprised," Warren explained. At that moment Morton arrived. He was out of breath and had obviously been running. He had been delayed in the completion of the apparatus which was used to administer the ether. Dr. Warren stepped back, indicated the man on the crude operating table and said, "Well, Sir, your patient is ready." Morton immediately applied the apparatus to the patient's mouth, advising him to breathe slowly and deeply and telling him that if he did so, he would quickly go to sleep. The patient eagerly responded to his instruction, and after breathing the vapor for about three minutes, sank into a deep state of insensibility. Morton looked up and said, "Dr. Warren, your patient is ready."

"Ready? When is anyone ever ready?" he thought. "I mean really ready. Never perhaps. What's good if it isn't a risk, and a risk means not being ready. It's the edge of things that count. That's where the scalpel is sharpest and that's where it cuts." He entered the room. The patient was by now anesthetized and had

been scrubbed by his assistants and draped by the nurses. He quickly gowned and gloved and then stepped to the table, his intern to the left, his resident directly opposite, the scrub nurse at the foot, all crowding in toward the bright red square of antiseptic-painted flesh peeking through the drapes, as if they were drawing closer to a fire for warmth. He asked for the first instrument, "Scalpel!"

He asked for the first instrument, "Scalpel!" The incredulous audience watched in stunned silence as he made the incision through the skin. The patient neither struggled nor cried out. He continued the operation and the tumor was removed. Still no sign of pain from the prostrate form lying quietly on the wooden operating table. The surgery completed, the wound sutured and dressings applied, Dr. Warren wiped his bloodied hands on a towel tendered by one of the nurses, and turning to the audience he said, "Gentlemen, this is no humbug!" He then left the room, followed by his entourage in the prescribed pecking order. Still asleep, the patient was wheeled out.

It had been three hours, but it had gone well. A little touchy around the abdominal aorta, but his fingers knew what they were doing. They belonged there. He knew it, and it seemed, so did the tumor. His scrub suit was sopping wet. He always sweated heavily when he operated. It was like spilling himself out, using himself up. He let his resident close the wound and left the operating room alone. He wanted to be by himself.

He wanted to be by himself and he sat on the hard bench in the first row until the other students had left, until the nurses had cleared away the bloodied instruments, the buckets of soiled dressings, the pink water which now filled the basins, until the porters had mopped the floor and had themselves left, closing the doors behind them, until the skylight was shuttered, until he was entirely alone. He reviewed in his mind the startling event he had been witness to. He was excited beyond containment, but of all the excitements he had ever known, this was the calmest because it was tempered by a fierce pride at being even a small part of the great gift given that morning.

He rose slowly from his seat and made his way to the stairs. He carefully descended to the ground floor and leaving the building, entered the busyness of a Boston morning. The sun was shining and he felt as if he had broken from a cloud. Friends called to him on the street, but he did not answer. He kept walking. He knew then that he would use himself up in his work, that he would always be walking, right to the edge, and beyond, and always alone.

Well, Hamlet couldn't have been written by a committee, and if you wanted to be honest about it, even the act of love was not two people, but rather one and one. And what could better tell what he had done that morning other than to describe it as an act of love. He stopped in the surgeon's lounge to have a cup of coffee. He joined the banter, but he was alone.

Epilogue

Soon after his demonstration of ether as an anesthetic, Morton joined in a bitter controversy with Dr. Charles Jackson of Boston and Dr. Crawford W. Long of Georgia to establish which of the three could claim priority for its use. For years an acrimonious and heated dispute raged to which Morton gave all his effort and funds, leaving him finally a saddened, embittered and impoverished man. At age 49, unrewarded and unacclaimed, he died. Jackson's hatred, jealousy and intrigue led him to attempted suicide and insanity. Long, considered a charlatan, lost his patent and ended his life, as did Morton and Jackson, rejected, resentful and alone.

Two Weeks Later

"**B**ut it's my right arm, you can't take it off."
Speaking is a fifteen-year-old Latino. His arm had been seriously mangled in an auto accident that wasn't his fault.

"That's the arm I used to win the fieldhouse ping-pong championship this year."

He also had serious fractures of both legs, but neither was as bad as the arm.

"I keep the trophy on the mantle at home. I look at it every night. I need the arm to polish it."

We performed a number of operations: a vein graft to the major artery which was torn, an open reduction and fixation of a fracture dislocation of the elbow, two unsuccessful attempts at skin grafting, extensive removal of gangrenous soft tissue...

Two weeks later we amputated the arm.

Corridor Scene

I'd like to get my case started. I have office hours at 10:00 and I haven't even made rounds. Sorry to hold you up. I had a breast biopsy, possible mastectomy, and it came back positive and infiltrating, so I had to do a radical. I hope I can break away by one o'clock. It's my afternoon off and I haven't played tennis this week. The second crew was up all night with that motorcycle accident. Two teenagers. I lost one after twelve pints of blood, and the second is in the ICU on a Bennett respirator, a tube in every opening and totally decerebrate. Speaking of "I see you," did you see the ass on that new blond nurse on three south? Speaking of ass, if I have to do another hemorrhoid, I'm going to switch to proctology, where I can indulge my anal fixation 100 percent of the time. You wouldn't joke about such things if you ever had it done to you. I did, and afterwards it feels like you're shitting razor blades for a week. Speaking of razor blades, did you hear about the nurse who tried to commit suicide by swallowing razor blades? She wasn't successful, but in the attempt she performed a tonsillectomy, appendectomy, and hemorrhoidectomy on herself and finally circumcised three interns. What's that buzzing noise? It's just another Code Blue signal. The team must be getting good. I understand they saved an 85 year-old man last week. Yes, indeed, but they broke all his ribs in the process and had to "trach" him afterwards. Now, that's what I call delaying death with dignity. Speaking of ribs, how about doubling for dinner Saturday night? Sounds good. Which restaurant? I don't know. What's your favorite dish? Without a doubt, Miss Houston on Five Northwest. No, seriously, where would you like to eat? At the Y, her Y. You're incorrigible. You're a slow operator. You're schizophrenic. So what if my id is a bit odd? Scalpel. Pain. Blood. Life. Laughs. Death. I can't stand nurses with runs in their stockings. I think I'll make it by one. Too bad about the radical. Only 35 years old and two kids. Boy, I sure need to work on my backhand.

Cinderella

She was an unmarried, 32-year-old woman who weighed more than 200 pounds.

"I'd like to have my feet fixed during my summer vacation. I have two weeks. Do you think that will be enough time?"

She worked in a bank and lived at home with her aging parents. She wanted her bunions corrected.

"I really can't afford to take off more time than that. I don't know how Mom and Dad will get along without me, even for the short period. I do all the cooking and house cleaning besides being the major breadwinner. They're really almost totally dependent on me."

He had been seeing her for years. Her parents were also his patients. It was true that they depended on her. They had complementary strokes, his on the right, hers on the left. However, what was equally true was her dependence on their dependency. Single and lonely, their need was the major justification for her life.

74

"Will my toes be straight after the operation? Do you think I'll be able to fit into petite shoes?"

She was looking for a miracle. Something that would alter her apparently hopeless future. After two weeks in the hospital she hoped that she would emerge a new person. It was a common fantasy. If she could only get a nose job, change her work, move to a new neighborhood, take off 50 pounds, find the right man, read the right book, get her feet fixed; any one of these or a hundred other similar acts that would make her a princess.

"I've always wanted good-looking feet." A faraway look veiled her eyes. "I know I'm overweight and have a poor complexion." She seemed to be speaking from somewhere outside the room. "At least, I could have pretty feet."

The glass slipper awaits.

Abbreviations

"**M**orning Rick, where you headed?"

"I'm off to the OR. Got a big schedule today, an Abd. hyst., three laps, two T and A's, a TUR, a head and a chest."

"Sounds exciting. How was last night in the ER?"

"Mash City, man, Mash City."

"Bad?"

"Not exactly good. It started out with two DOAs and then a high FUO."

"Those can be interesting. What did you order?"

"The usual, SMA-12, CBC, EKG, BMR, Lytes."

"Did you get an LP?"

"No, I wasn't interested in the CSF."

"Any x-rays?"

"A chest and a stat KUB. No evidence of TB or VD."

"What were the findings?"

"Not much, just a fever, a split SI and URI, not even GC."

"What did you do with it?"

"Sent it to the ICU."

"So, what else?"

"Next we had a decomp."

"Did you dij him?"

"After the MS, of course, b.i.d. By the way, how's your GSW in 415?"

"Doing fine. He went off IVs and started on OT and PT yesterday. Rick, you ought to be getting tired of all this cutting and sewing. What's your next service?"

"OB - GYN next, then GI, then ENT. Just can't wait to get through all the LOAs and ROAs."

"Well, don't lose faith, another six months and you'll be done. So long, Rick, see you in the OR in the A.M."

"Or the ER in the P.M."

❈

The Seamstress

Her daughter explained, "She's an old seamstress, Doctor, you know how they say in Yiddish, 'A tapton a schtickele ware.' She has a need to touch the material."

"I understand, but if she can't keep her hands from under the dressing, the sore will never heal."

There was a varicose ulcer on her leg which she insisted on scratching.

"I wish I could cooperate better, Doctor." She is talking now, 75 years old, living by herself, her only companions pain, loneliness and a varicose ulcer.

"It itches, so of course I scratch it. And then, just every once in awhile, I like to take a peek to see how well it's healing. The itching means it's healing, nu?"

How could he be upset with her? They were both old seam-stresses under the skin. She only in a figurative sense; he literally. For he, too, had the need to be forever touching flesh, the ultimate fabric.

He put her in a plaster cast, hoping to keep her curious fingers away from the leg, at least until it healed.

"A tapton a schtickele ware," indeed!

Scrub Talk

"**Y**ou look tired."

"I am tired. I was up all night."

"Not with me you weren't."

"No, if you remember, that was last week. Steinhauer's hernia kept me up last night."

"Strangulated?"

"You bet. His ruptures give me a pain in the groin!"

"Why didn't he do it yesterday afternoon? Didn't he think it would strangulate?"

"Apparently not, besides he had a golf date. He's a comer, that Steinhauer is."

"That's no way to talk about your chief."

"He's been making the same mistakes for twenty years, only now he calls it experience."

"Look who's talking, you haven't even had your first mal-practice suit."

"Now Marge, don't poor-mouth me, I've had lots of experi-ence ..."

"Yeah, I know, if you have one case, you say, 'In my experi-ence ...'; if you have two cases, you say, "In my series ...'" and if you have three, it's "In case after case after case ... '".

"Want to know a secret?"

"You know I never encourage hospital gossip. I think it's cruel and unfair. Tell me quick!"

"He wears a truss."

"Who wears a truss?"

"Steinhauer, who else!"

"You're putting me on."

"I swear by Apollo! And Marge, you wouldn't believe it, there are more trusses in that surgeons' locker room than there are jockstraps on the first string of the Chicago Bears."

"Why, that sissy, won't submit to the knife, eh?"

"Ain't it a shame."

"I think we've scrubbed ten minutes."

"Must be, my fingernails are starting to bleed."

"Isn't this your case?"

"It's nothing really, just a little stump revision I slipped in between my majors."

"Minor surgery, my dear, is an operation performed on someone else. Besides, as far as I can remember, you've never been scheduled for one of these before. How come so cocky?"

"See one, do one, teach one."

"Well, let's go. The sooner I get started, the sooner I get off my bunions."

"Your feet hurt? Want to lie down? Well then, how about staying up all night with me? I can't promise you a strangulated hernia, but ..."

"You're a fast operator, Doctor, but my cats would object. Besides, I'm in love with my work and I take Geritol. Try the student nurse in Operating Room 6. She's more your type."

"O.K. Marge, no harm in asking. The wish isn't the act."

"Just keep your hands off my Mayo stand and we'll stay friends."

"Friends it is, Marge."

"A truss, eh? Can you feature that? What a rascal!"

Surgery

Dealing Dan the Bargain Man

There's a joker in every pack.

"I'm the oldest son, so the family elected me spokesman. How bad is she, doctor?"

"Your mother has a broken hip. We have to operate to put it back together and hold it with a pin and plate. With proper care and barring complications, she should be up in a chair the day after surgery and walking with a cane shortly after that."

"Is there any danger?"

"I don't anticipate any unusual problems, but she is 75 years old and will have to be watched very closely. Her internist, Dr. Green, is running some tests. He'll let me know when we can schedule surgery."

"All she has is her government insurance; what will this whole deal cost?"

"My average fee in these cases is $2,000 and Medicare usually covers most of that. Why don't we wait and see what the insurance pays, I can always make an adjustment on the balance. I don't want to impose a financial hardship on you."

"But how about the cost of the hospital and her internist's fee?"

"You'll have to discuss that with the business office and Dr. Green. I'm sure they'll be considerate of your means."

"Do you think we could get this done cheaper elsewhere?"

"I don't know. You could try, but we keep a close tab on our charges. I assure you they're average or even below average for this area."

"Does your quote include all the extras? Taking out the stitches? Visits to your office? The cane and so forth?"

"Well, everything she'll need in the way of service is included. As far as appliances, that will entail a small additional charge."

"Maybe we could make a deal for you to just take the insurance, and that's all. How about it, Doc?"

"As I said, I don't intend to place a burden on you. I promise to be very reasonable about the fee. Let's just get her well and see what the insurance pays."

"O.K. Doc, you sound straight to me. But no offense if I ask around a bit?"

"Of course not, no offense at all."

"Good, glad you see it my way. Well, I'll call you later this afternoon and let you know what I decide. You know my name and if you have to get hold of me, I can be reached at this number. It's my place of business, 'South Suburban Used Cars, the Hottest Deal in Town.' Just ask for 'Dealing Dan', that's me. By the way, Doc, you're not in the market for a good used car, are you?"

Tincture of Time

As the old tinsmith used to say, "You measure ten times and then you cut once."

"I want an operation. I'm sure it would help."

"I'm not certain surgery is indicated in your case. I'd like to run a few more tests."

"But just a few months ago I read in the *Reader's Digest* that 90 percent of people with my condition are helped by an operation."

"And if you're one of the 10 percent that's not helped?"

"Ninety to 10 is pretty good odds."

"But if you're one of the 10, it's 100 percent for you."

"Nonetheless, I'd like to try."

"I'm not saying we won't eventually operate. I just want to make absolutely certain of the need to do so. It's easy enough to cut, but I haven't as yet found a way to uncut. There's no orthopedic condition that the wrong operation can't make worse. Just a bit more patience; a little more tincture of time."

"What's that?"

"It's time in a bottle, to be taken as advised."

"But that's silly and besides it's impossible."

"Silly? Impossible? It's not and I wish it weren't."

As the old tinsmith said, "You measure ten times and then you cut once."

Chop! Chop!

Okay, let's move. Chop! Chop!
Towels.

That's it, get the sheets in place.

Raise the table about two inches and adjust the light, please.

Are we ready?

Scalpel.

Sponge.

Hemostat.

Another.

Another.

Another.

Okay, let's tie.

Second knife.

Rake retractors.

Scissors.

No, I prefer the heavy Mayo.

Nice.

Hemostat.

Catch that one now.

Got it?

Good.
Stick tie.
Scissors again.
Deep retractors.
Periosteal elevator.
There it is.
Give me a little traction.
Bone holder.
Just a little more rotation, please.
Hold that now.
Damn it, it slipped!
Once again.
Now hold it this time.
That's it. Tighten the clamp.
I think it'll take a 3-inch plate.
Drill.
Depth gauge.
Screwdriver.
1½ inch screws.
Another ... another ... another.
That ought to hold it.
Okay, close it in layers, no drain, the usual dressing.
Write post-op orders for me, will you? I'll start rounds.
Thanks everyone.
Good job!

DEATH

I visit your bedside as a fellow prisoner because we are all condemned to death. I come to tell you that I understand, for I myself am also afraid. I will not be hypocritical with you. I do not know if there is life after death. What I do know is that hospital life is often played out like a Greek tragedy, where most of the turmoil occurs off stage. But there need be no turmoil in this process, particularly if it is shared. Besides, in conscience, I could not protect you from it if I wished. I could only protect myself. And that, in fact, is the problem I face. In denying your death, I deny my own. In refusing to recognize your loneliness, your fear, your need, I repress my own. You see, it is really very selfish of me; for if I cannot permit you to die consciously and with dignity, I cannot live consciously and with dignity. Therefore, I visit your bedside as a fellow prisoner, and I accept us exactly as we are — afraid, alone, and in need. In all our perfection.

❖

Balancing

He had noticed an interesting clinical correlation. As the body wastes, the eyes enlarge, or so it seemed. He had discovered this during his worst time, Thursday afternoons. This is when he held the Muscle Disease Clinic.

He usually saw ten to fifteen such patients, for whose affliction there was no known cause or cure, slowly dying, a little weaker each visit, their limbs wasting and their eyes enlarging, until they swallowed him in their futile hope.

Try as he might, he could not balance in himself the tensions these Thursday afternoons created. Most of these clinic patients were children with muscular dystrophy, destined for a wheelchair in their early teens and death before twenty, and he often wondered if he would ever lose the courage to continue to fail in their behalf.

He had tried to learn everything he could about the disease, so as to offer his patients the best treatment available. He knew that his skills had significantly increased their function and comfort and may have even somewhat lengthened their life expectancy. But even knowing this didn't help him. Not for long, anyway.

For a time he made a habit of having dinner out, followed by a movie or other entertainment on Thursday nights. This, too, didn't help. Next, he tried drinking in the evening. He couldn't get drunk, he only got sick. Finally, he decided to visit the YMCA on the way home from the clinic to jog or to swim. He also began carrying his skates in the car, stopping at an indoor ice rink for an hour or so. He wasn't particularly adept at any of these things, but the motor release was good for him. He didn't have to think, only move.

While running he would close his eyes and swing his arms, savoring the feeling of his own healthy muscles stretching and straining. In the pool he would kick and pull, breathing regularly, back and forth, back and forth, allowing the water to slowly dilute his tensions. He liked the ice skating best of all. The swiftness of it appealed to him. Also, the anxiety of being slightly off-balance and having to quickly regain equilibrium. The sensation of controlling stabilization, which is what ice skating is all about, was reassuring to him. Round and round the rink he would skate, feeling his body swing in rhythmic stride, faster, yet faster. Clenching his teeth against the scream rising in his throat. On balance, then off balance, on balance, then off balance, on balance ... then off balance ... on balance ... off balance ... on ... off ...

The Question

She was 92 years old and slowly bleeding out from a peptic ulcer. The question was should we transfuse her. She said, "Holy Mary, Mother of God." That's what she said, just that, "Holy Mary, Mother of God," and she kept saying it over and over again. She was 92 and slowly bleeding out from an ulcer. She had not walked in ten years. She was incontinent of urine and stool. She was blind and half deaf. The question was should she be transfused.

All old people smell the same. My parents are beginning to smell like my grandparents smelled. No doubt, some day, I too will smell the same. They smell like the hallway to their apartment smells. The apartment smells like they do. Everything smells the same, my grandparents, my parents, their apartment, and the hallway. If we live long enough, we'll all smell the same —we'll smell like that hallway.

She was brought into the emergency room as an overdose. She was over 90. She lived in a nursing home. She had a bed, a chair, a bedside table, and half a closet. The other half was for her roommate whose portion of the room could be separated for privacy from hers by a curtain which ran on a track in the ceiling. She kept her few personal effects in a brown paper bag. She had saved her sleeping medication for two weeks and then taken it all at once.

She smelled like my grandmother, or the hallway to my parents' apartment. The question is, should she be resuscitated?

The real question is, how much is too much? I once saw a family abandon an older member (mother? grandmother? aunt?) simply by placing her on a cart in the emergency room corridor and leaving, something like abandoning a baby on the doorstep. "Here, we can't handle this any longer. It's too much. You take over." They ran and I pursued. They soon outdistanced me, of course. They ran faster. Their need was more desperate than mine.

Do you know where you are? What day is it? Who's the President of the United States? They get smaller, the old ones. As the room becomes more and more cluttered with life-sustaining appliances, they seem to get smaller and smaller, until they are gone and only the pain is left. Everything comes full circle. And the old man, surrounded by strange equipment he doesn't understand, asking questions he cannot answer, feeling feelings he cannot explain; scared like a helpless little boy, comes finally to die in his childhood.

"I'm sorry to be dying, Doctor. I know it embarrasses you, but I'm very tired. I have this tube in my throat. I can't speak and I have to tell you all this with my eyes. You see, I have this disease. It's caused me to become very weak, weak to the point where I can no longer breathe by myself. And now I have this tube in my throat. The tube is connected to a pipe, and the pipe is connected to a machine. The machine is plugged into the wall, where electricity makes it work. It's a sort of pump and it breathes for me. I can never leave the bed because I'm attached to the machine. Each day I get weaker. I'm so weak I can't move, I just lie here. But the machine is very much alive. It is in fact more alive than I am. I know I'm dying, Doctor, and I apologize for the inconvenience."

The question is, who will pull the plug?

The question is, "Holy Mary, Mother of God"— the question is, "What is the question?"

※

Jenny

She is eighty years old.
"I can't stand to look how he's dying."

Her name is Jenny.

"He wasn't just a doctor, also a dear friend he was." She's crying. "I can't get it over from him to see how he's wasting away." Like a child, frightened.

"He's so kind, he takes care of people." Hands wringing a lace handkerchief.

"For years he's known us, like one of the family." Her moist eyes magnified by thick lenses.

"He'd hold my hand when I was sick, so patient he was." Antique broach closing her dress at the neck.

"I'd rather I would go."

Silence now.

Sobbing without restraint.

"I'd

rather

I

would

go."

※

We Are All

I went to the funeral.
"It was nice of you to come."

"I did everything I could."

He was lying quietly in his coffin.

O Gentlest Heart of Jesus, ever present in the Blessed Sacrament, ever consumed with burning love for the poor captive souls in Purgatory, have mercy on the soul of Thy departed servant.

"We know you did everything you could."

Yes, I did everything I could.

Be not severe in Thy judgment but let some drops of Thy Precious Blood fall upon the devouring flames.

I went to the funeral.

"It was nice of his class to come. The sister gave them the afternoon off so they could come as a class. They said a Hail Mary for him. It was very nice of them to come. It was very nice of them to say a Hail Mary."

And to Thou O Merciful Savior send Thy angels to conduct Thy departed servant to a place of refreshment, light and peace.

"He was only twelve years old, but he suffered so. And now he is finally at peace."

We are all trapped in our own heads.

Lord Jesus, the one hope of my salvation.

We are all ...

Autopsy Scene

Stinks and sights. Sewer and toilet smells. Sharp stink of formalin. Salty smell of blood. Butcher shop smells. Blue smell of veins, white smell of nerves. Bright colors — yellow of fat, hard glisten of bone, foamy gray color of lungs, strong dusky red of heart filled with grape jelly purple clots. Thin, almost transparent small intestine, glistening liver capsule and turgid spleen. Chicken guts. Empty body. Headless. Pieces into bottles. Life into bottles. Life into machines. Death ... nothing special ... only death.

The Dream

It was the same dream. It never changed. He just dreamt it more frequently now.

In the dream he could choose his own death from those of the patients he had attended, but was unable to help. So, he walked through his past like some sick zoo, witnessing again the violence and the final agony of all those he could not save.

The young girl who fell from her fifteenth story apartment. The high school football player who died of an overdose. The suicides of every variety, slashed wrists, poisonings, gunshot wounds. The full vocabulary of self-inflicted hate. The road accidents. The drownings. The stabbings. The stillbirths. The stranglings and the gaspings. The tumors and the clots. The cruel deaths and the quiet ones. The young, the old. And, oh yes, the children and the drunks. Always, the children and the drunks.

He saw them all, but at the end of the thought tunnel he finally realized there was no choice. He was ultimately his own executioner, and whatever dying was given him, he would long before choke to death on his own hope.

He abruptly awoke in a cold sweat, to stare into the darkness and listen again to the silence.

Fairy Tale

Once upon a time there lived a brave king and his fair queen. They had a little princess who was an albino; so fair was she that everyone called her "Snow White."

One day the queen died of typhoid fever, a disease common in those times of outside plumbing and poor castle sanitation.

The king, in his despair, took to wife a psychopathic sadist (with a mirror fetish) who, jealous of her stepdaughter, drove her from the castle.

Snow White wandered for days in the evil forest until, lost and exhausted, she fell asleep.

When she awakened, she was startled to find herself at the home of the seven dwarfs. With eagerness she cleaned the house and prepared dinner, anticipating their return from work. When they finally arrived, she couldn't believe her eyes.

Expecting to see Sleepy, Bashful, Grumpy, Happy, Sneezy, Dopey and Doc, she was instead faced with seven real dwarfs: one of the hypothalamic pituitary type; another a stunted achondroplastic; the third a dull cretin; the fourth a failure-to-thrive infant; the fifth a case of diastrophic dwarfism, complicated by diabetes insipidus and adrenal insuffiency; the sixth a leprechaun; and the seventh a Morquio's syndrome.

Snow White suddenly realized that in truth Sleeping Beauty had narcolepsy and will never awaken; beauty is beauty, beast is always beast; Rapunzel had dandruff and Cinderella delusions; and no matter how many frogs you kiss, not a one ever turns into a handsome prince. Only in the wonderful world of Disney are the seven dwarfs cuddly and cute. In real life, they are sick and sad.

Thus, poor, little, disillusioned Snow White ran screaming from the cottage of the seven dwarfs into the blackness of the night, from where she was never heard of again.

And nobody lived happily ever after.

Because there is no ever after.

I'd Walk Away

"I don't wanna die, Doctor, I don't wanna die."

"It's a scary thought, Debbie, I know it's a scary thought."

"It's not that I'm scared, Doctor. I'm sort of, well, I'm sort of ashamed."

"There's nothing at all to be ashamed of, Debbie. Nothing that's happened to you has in any way been your fault."

"I'll miss you when I die, Doctor. I'll miss you when I die."

"I feel very close to you too, Debbie. I feel like neither of us is alone."

"But I want to walk, Doctor. If I could just walk before I die."

"If I could make you walk, you know I would, Debbie."

"The other night I dreamed that I walked, Doctor. The other night I dreamed that I got out of my wheelchair and walked. If I could just do that when I wasn't dreaming, you know what I'd do?"

"What would you do Debbie?"

"I'd walk away, Doctor. I'd walk away so fast even death would never catch up with me."

Shirley, Age 47

Shirley, age 47, her skeleton weakened by tumor metastasis, kept breaking bones. It all started when she had her tonsils irradiated as a child, a then in vogue treatment for tonsillitis, a benign condition. Unfortunately, her thyroid, a gland not far from the tonsils, was also irradiated and underwent malignant change.

91

In spite of the deadly flower carrying her death message which began to grow there, she managed, with radical surgery, chemotherapy, and other lifesaving measures, to keep it all together long enough to tend house and raise a family. Now, the tumor had reached and weakened her bones, and they were breaking one by one. First her right arm. Then her right thigh. Then her left pelvis. What next, Shirley, what next? Her vital organs weren't as yet seriously involved, so Shirley is very much alive in spite of the fact that the least false move or undue pressure breaks yet another bone. What to do, what to do? An operation here, some traction there, perhaps a cast or two. How long can you keep this up, Shirley? When will you throw in the sponge? Why don't you die, Shirley? Quietly, the way you're supposed to, you know what I mean, without any fuss. Why can't you act as we expect any self-respecting patient with cancer to perform? You know, Shirley, it's beginning to annoy us. You're getting on our nerves. I can't cure you, and I certainly can't kill you. Accept the facts of life (and death), Shirley. Is it really worth the trouble? Come now, Shirley, be reasonable. Each time you break a bone, you break my heart a little more. Even if you have the strength to take it, I don't think I can last much longer.

Ginah

"A surgeon always walks with fear," he remembered the old maxim, "fear for his mistakes, fear for his shortcomings, but never fear for his reputation, never fear for himself." But here in Java, where he was volunteering a month of service, he had no reputation, and as far as what constituted his self, he had no idea.

"Twan (boss)," Harsano, his driver, pointed out to him one day in Pidgin English while they were locked in a traffic jam of Asian proportions. "There are three many people here for comfort." "Three many" sometimes took on a comic aspect, as when he made ward rounds and discovered two giggling faces in the same bed. This never turned out to be a janiceps monster, just a couple of sick kids helping to solve the overcrowding by sharing sheets. It was all quite extraordinary, but he had come to the Far East with the notion that one way of understanding the ordinary was to understand the extraordinary; or was it that everything was extraordinary, or maybe nothing. He didn't know, yet.

Her name was Ginah. She was coming to the city for market. The train, as usual, was dirty and slow, with many passengers crowding its platforms and clinging to its sides in a futile attempt to escape the crush and the heat inside. Ginah was one of these. The ancient steam engine tugged and rattled its human cargo down the jungle track, and Ginah lost her grip and slipped between the wheels.

He first saw her in the receiving room. Her right leg had been amputated above the knee and her right arm above the elbow. There was no blood bank at the hospital, and the clinic was ill-equipped for a procedure of this magnitude. Ginah was only 28 years old. He would try.

He was used to working in the tropical heat. He had even accustomed himself to the ill fitting surgical gowns, the shredding suture, the ancient instruments, and the heavy rubber gloves re-sterilized so many times that they often fell apart when touched. What was still odd to him was operating in bare feet, a practice maintained for comfort and supposed cleanliness. Working fast, he cleaned, revised, and closed the amputation sites. At one point he felt something wet trickle to his feet. He knew what it was, but looked anyway. It was Ginah's blood ... it felt warm.

She died late that afternoon. The nurse told him that she had said she no longer wanted to live, as she would be a burden to her family and because she had lost her right hand. In the Muslim faith — he was told — it is taboo to eat with the left hand, as it is used to clean oneself at toilet. He did not know whether or not to believe she had said this. He knew the Javanese were stoical, even fatalistic, and death had a different meaning for them than for Westerners. He remembered something another patient had once said to him after he had spent most of the night saving a mangled limb. "Doctor," he said, "I am glad for you." But Ginah was no longer glad for him, if indeed she had ever been, nor was he at that moment very glad for himself.

It was the season of the monsoon, and that evening he awakened to the thunder of an oncoming storm, mixing with the drone of the ceiling fan. He arose, naked and slick with sweat. He walked to the louvered French doors and, opening them, stepped onto the balcony. The sky was darkening and the first drops of tropical rain had already begun to softly fall. They struck his head and trickled down to this feet. He noticed that where the rain touched his body, it was warm. It then occurred to him that from the very first he had known he could not save her, but that he must try, because his life, in a curious way, as well as hers also seemed to be at stake. He had always taken for granted that his patients valued life to the same degree and in the same way as he. And now he had failed, for death, to him, was the ultimate failure. But for Ginah, the problem had been both created and solved when the train ran over her, for the idea of living as she had been left was as intolerable to her as the idea of her dying was to him. Everyone else at the hospital knew this, and the rest was a charade for his benefit alone.

Recognizing that he, too, was the object of his grief, he felt a sudden emptiness, as if someone was walking over his grave. Though it was as yet unresolved in his rational mind, he realized that he had to come to terms with his fear. Standing there on the balcony, he gave himself permission to mourn both Ginah's death and his own ... as the sky continued to darken and the storm drew near.

The Comedian

The comedian limped onto the stage on crutches.

"A funny thing happened to me on the way to the hospital," he began.

The audience roared. He then told two jokes. One had to do with bleeding during major surgery and the other with the problems of using a bedpan on an intensive care unit. Next, he imitated a spastic. It was very funny.

"And now it's time to play The Newly-Dead Game," he bantered.

He did a soft shoe dance number which mimicked a triple amputee, sang two requests, "The song is over, but the malady lingers on" and "Please give me something to dismember you by," and finished up by performing a pseudo-epileptic fit.

The audience loved him. He was the best comedian the hospital ever had. So good in fact that all other acts were canceled; the magician who restored eyesight and lost hearing, the armless acrobat, the voiceless chorus, the sightless sharpshooting rifle team, the legless high-jumpers, even the thalidomide babies clapping their flippers and begging for more thalidomide, and only the comedian was booked for the duration.

The hospital administration went to his dressing room to tell him the good news. He didn't answer when they knocked on the door. They broke it down and found the comedian dead, his now aged face smeared with roses and streaked with tears, his wasted body wounded by the sharp edges of the darkness in which he moved all his life.

The coroner's report said simply that he had cried himself to death.

Have a Nice Day

She had malignant disease. This was her third operation. It was a perfect spring day. As he turned to leave following his morning visit, she looked at him, smiled, and said:

"G'bye, Doctor, have a nice day."

The hospital visitors' elevator was crowded, but the well-dressed elderly man managed to squeeze himself in. As the lift began its ascent, the elevator's occupants announced their floors to the operator. After everyone, except he, had announced his floor, the operator turned to the gentleman and politely inquired, "And what floor would you like, Sir?"

He stood bemused for a few seconds, and then turning to the others on board and without cracking a smile asked, "Today is Saturday, isn't it?"

"Yes," several passengers volunteered.

"Then I'll take the sixth floor!" he stated emphatically.

"G'bye, Doctor, have a nice day."

"How long have you had this pain, Mrs. Weinstein?"

"It feels numb in my legs, mostly the right."

"Where does it hurt the most?"

"I've had it for about two months."

"Did it start suddenly or come about slowly?"

"It hurts mostly in the ankles."

"Is it ever relieved by rest, or is it present all the time?"

"It came on gradually."

"Does weather seem to affect it?"

"Sometimes it's better if I lie down."

"But does weather seem to affect it?"

"But like I said, my legs are numb."

"G'bye, Doctor, have a nice day."

"I used to be a beauty, Doctor. Fair skin, golden tresses, and, oh, my beautiful eyes. They used to say of me, 'With my pupils, I should be a teacher.'"

"G'bye, Doctor, have a nice day."

"I can't move my arm. Does that mean I've got an icy shoulder?"

"I got hit in the eye with a handball. I can't see very well. I hope I don't have a hemorrhoid in the eye."

"G'bye, Doctor, have a nice day."

"G'bye, Doctor, have a nice day."

"G'bye, Doctor, have a nice"

"G'bye, Doctor, have a"

"G'bye, Doctor"

"G'bye."

Just Like That

He was a doctor, not very old, and in apparent good health. Nonetheless, he died of a myocardial infarct. And he died very quickly; a sudden pain in the chest and then he was gone. Just like that.

His colleagues were stunned. Everyone at the hospital talked a little more softly at breakfast the next morning. And no doubt they all hugged their kids a bit harder when tucking them in; they were less hurried on morning rounds; and several even swore off cigarettes for the umpteenth time. Those who had suffered heart attacks and recovered were especially perturbed. Rumors flew free and wild.

"He had severe diabetes that he was treating himself. No one else knew about it."

"His family history was terrible. Two brothers died of heart trouble before the age of 40."

"This was his third attack. The other two were minor episodes that he ignored. Besides, he'd been walking around for three days with chest pain, but wouldn't stop to take an ECG."

Thus consoled, they went back to checking their own pulses.

But all of these things were untrue. The fact was that he died, even though he was a doctor. A sudden pain in the chest and then he was gone. Just like that.

❖

I'll Have to Sleep On It

"We know it's near the end, but we don't want him to die, not yet, please Doctor, not yet." A mother is speaking. Her 16-year-old son, suffering from muscular dystrophy and wheelchair bound, has been admitted through the emergency room in severe respiratory distress. A tube was inserted into his trachea, but he can't breathe without assistance and is now in the ICU attached to a respirator.

"We'll do everything we can, Mrs. Bosworth, everything we can."

"Every time I look at him and see how weak he's getting, and know how difficult it is for him to do the simplest things, like feed himself, or even swallow, I wish very quietly and very deep inside myself, that some morning he might not wake up, and all the fear and all the waiting would be over for both of us."

Another mother, another youngster with muscular dystrophy, another hope, albeit different, equally agonized, equally honest.

"His sisters miss him so much at home."

"I'm sure he's thought of it even though he hasn't said anything."

"His birthday is in another month."

"It breaks my heart to see him struggle so."

98

"He can't talk on the machine, but his eyes tell me that he wants to live."

"Isn't there a way to end this quickly, without pain?"

"When will they find the cause? The cure?"

"There's is no cure."

"Don't let him die."

"Why doesn't he die?"

Not to die. Ought to die.

I don't know the answer. I'll have to sleep on it. Give me a hundred years or so.

PATIENTS

Why this fascination with disease? Is it truly, as the psychoanalysts say, a way of mastering our own fears of mutilation and death? "Gnothi Seauton" is the inscription at Delphi. "Know thyself," for that knowing holds if not the important answers, at least the important questions. This is the ideal. To put one's mind over what matters. To see illness and cure, suffering and healing, as a single, common human experience. As complementary parts of the same process, as are men and women, as are day and night, as are life and death. A doctor and his patient are not so different after all. They have the same needs, they seek the same goal. The word "patient" means to bear with composure. Is this not what the physician most also do? The word "doctor" derives from the Latin, "docere," to teach, and this is what a patient always does if his doctor will but allow him. A doctor doesn't treat a patient, nor is a patient the passive recipient of the physician's ministrations. They are actively bound in a mutual cause. Much like lovers. For medicine is after all best practiced as a form of love.

A Ziegfeld Girl

Through the thick lenses her eyes appeared strangely out of proportion with the rest of her face. Yet, they were attractive in a sad brown way, as if she had purposely contrived to magnify what little remained of the long-faded beauty of her youth.

And once she had been beautiful indeed. She even displayed an old scrapbook whose yellowed clippings certified the fact that she had once danced in the Ziegfeld chorus. But she was now seventy years old, living alone in a small room in a seedy neighborhood, and she wore thick lenses in a desperate attempt to aid her cataracted eyes.

"I got up at night to use the washroom ... I had misplaced my glasses, but thought I knew the way well enough not to need them .. I reached for the light cord and tripped ... The cord was too short anyway, and the fluorescent light flickers when you turn it on ... My landlord is such a 'Gonif' ... He won't replace anything that's broken ... The faucet drips and the toilet leaks ... This is the third time I stumbled at home this week ... The front step is cracked and I tripped on that two days ago ... I skinned my knee badly ... I could have broken my head ... He doesn't give us enough heat in the winter, and my room is stifling during the summer because I can't afford an air conditioner ... He keeps promising to make necessary repairs, but all he does is lie, lie, lie ... The housing office is no help, and my Social Security check is so small I can't afford to move elsewhere ... My diabetes is worse and I'm slowly going blind ... It doesn't matter, though ... I've seen all there is to see, the good and the bad, there's really nothing else left for me to see anymore ..."

Her eyes so filled the room, I was forced to close my own.

Bible Lesson

There is an old Yiddish joke that goes:

Question: "What does a Rabbi send his doctor for Chanukah?"

Answer: "Another Rabbi!"

Some of the myth of his service to Israel had spilled out of the medical and into the religious community, and a number of rabbis sought his consultation. He enjoyed them, especially the Hassidic group. Fanatics, particularly fundamentalists, interested him because he had no answers and was always intrigued by anyone claiming to have them all. They were, however, a difficult group to attend, but he had his own tricks.

"So Nu? What's the diagnosis?" The Rabbi was 50 and looked 60. His shoulders stooped from hours of study, but his eyes were bright, even mischievous, as he stroked his beard with dignified talmudic concern.

"Nothing serious, Rabbi, only a little degenerative arthritis of the knee."

"And what's the treatment?" he asked, adjusting his black skull cap.

"Again, nothing spectacular. Some strengthening exercises, aspirin for pain, local heat, avoid strain, and, by all means, lose weight."

"And when will it get better?" This with a finger to the forehead.

"I can't say, Rabbi. We just have to wait and see."

"So what kind of a doctor can't give me some idea how long I'll have to suffer?" This with the palms outstretched and the eyes rolled toward the ceiling.

"Rabbi."

"Yes?"

"Do you recall that in the book of Genesis, the Lord instructed Adam that he might partake of the fruit of any tree in the garden of Eden, but cautioned him not to eat the fruit of the tree of the knowledge of good and evil?"

"Yes, of course. He warned him that if he ate of the fruit of the tree of the knowledge of good and evil, he would surely die."

"Correct. And did Adam eat of that fruit?"

"You know he did."

"And how long did Adam live after that?"

"The Bible says he lived over 600 years."

"Well, Rabbi, if God himself can't give an accurate prognosis in the case of Adam's life expectancy, how do you expect me to give one in the case of your knee!"

So Far

When a mother is the only adult accompanying the child on an office visit, it is usually the child's problem, occasionally the mother's. When the grandmother arranges the visit and comes along, it is usually her problem, often the mother's, and seldom the child's.

"She's 11½ months old and hasn't walked yet. Her mother was running by that time. There must be something wrong!"

Grandma is speaking. She is carefully cosmetized to camouflage her 65 years. The hair tint is of dubious success.

"As I've told you before, she's a perfectly normal child, and right on time as far as motor development is concerned."

"I don't like the way she has of holding on when she stands. She seems so unsure of herself. Are you certain there's nothing wrong?"

"It's perfectly normal for an 11-month-old to hold onto something for support when first learning to walk. Besides, she's not only your daughter's first child, but also the family's first grandchild. I suspect that everyone waits on her hand and foot, and she's not given the opportunity to walk much."

"I don't know why you say that, Doctor. It's true I'm at Thelma's apartment four or five times a week, but after all, I'm there to help. And it's no easy chore to raise a child. I know, I raised one myself."

"I wasn't implying anything, Mrs. Rosen, I was just trying to reassure you."

I've affronted her, and for this I'm sorry. She has been widowed many years. My pique melts to pity.

"I was the one," she continues, "who took care of the baby from the moment she left the hospital. It is my training that will get her on the potty before she's two. So of course I'm concerned about her welfare."

I look at the beautiful, normal, healthy child before me, not quite knowing what to say next.

So far, the mother hasn't uttered a word.

It Seems Like

"What's the trouble?"

"It seems like I've got a pain in my right shoulder."

"How long have you had it?"

"It seems like it's been there at least a month, maybe two."

"How did it start? Did you injure yourself in any way?"

"No, I didn't fall or anything like that. It seems like it was just there when I woke up one morning."

"Do you have the pain all the time?"

"It seems like it never goes away."

"Does anything make it worse or make it better?"

"It seems like using the arm makes it worse and a hot bath makes it better."

"Well, take off your shirt, sit up on the examining table, and I'll take a look."

"What do you think it is?"

"Well now, I can't say for sure until after I've examined you and we'll probably need some x-rays. But it seems to me like you've got 'seems like' disease."

※

Just Fine

There won't be any more like them after their generation passes. You know the type. They immigrated to America at the turn of the century, lived in a ghetto, speaking mostly Yiddish, worked 60 hours a week at a menial trade or small business, mending, making do. They saved every penny, so their children would have all the opportunities. Children who now practice professions, live in the suburbs, and play golf at fancy country clubs.

He wears the jacket from one suit, the pants from another. Her old dress is graced with a filigreed antique brooch. They have only their social security, but refuse clinic care. They are as tender to each other as two gentle children at quiet play.

Holding hands for support, they slowly enter my examining room, out of some strange pride, refusing to use the canes I recommended.

"How are you today, Mrs. Schwartz? And you, Samuel, how do you feel?"

"Just fine, Doctor. Just fine. But you look a little tired. You really should slow down and take better care of yourself."

I Make a Living

"I have a pain in my Semitic nerve."

"In your what?"

"In my Semitic nerve. You know, the one that Jacob injured when he was struggling with the angel. I guess you call it the sciatic nerve. I call it the Semitic nerve."

"And were you also injured struggling with an angel?"

"No, I wasn't struggling with anyone. I think I got it from sitting in a cab twelve hours at a stretch. I drive a yellow hack in Chicago."

"Isn't that a tough job for a seventy-year-old?"

"I've got to feed myself."

"Do you have a wife? Children?"

"I lost them all when I left Germany in 1937."

"So you live alone?"

"I live with my sister and her husband."

"Why do you think the cab driving has something to do with the sciatica, excuse me, Semitica?"

"Have you ever bounced in a cab for twelve hours a day? It's 'schwere Arbeit,' 'Schwarze' work."

"Did you try taking some time off, soaking in a hot tub, resting?"

"I did that the last few days."

"So, how are you doing?"

"Nu, I make a living."

◼

Deposition

"Tell me what happened?"

"On or about May 5th, at approximately 4:30 in the afternoon, I tripped on a broken sidewalk at the northeast corner of Monroe and Dearborn Streets, falling and sustaining injuries to my back and legs."

"And after you fell?"

"I was taken by a police ambulance to the nearest hospital where x-rays were taken."

"What did the x-rays show?"

"The x-rays were negative for fracture, but examination at that time revealed extensive soft tissue injuries."

"And then?"

"I asked to be hospitalized, but was told there were no beds available. I therefore took a taxi home, placed myself in bed, and called my personal physician."

"What did he do?"

"He prescribed a narcotic for pain, a sedative for sleep, local heat for my back, and suggested I consult an orthopedic surgeon for further treatment."

"Have you ever had trouble with your back or legs before?"

"Prior to the aforesaid accident I have had only occasional, transient back distress which never required bed rest."

"Do you feel that your recent injury aggravated your previous back condition?"

"It could or might have."

"By the way, what do you do for a living?"

"I'm an attorney."

"I thought that was likely."

"What made you think so?"

"Well, on or about the second question you answered I began to get that idea, but the aforementioned feeling could or might have just been my intuition."

Holiday Syndrome

I call it the holiday syndrome.

"It's a 'paint' in mine back and I get weak in mine legs."

She raised a family. Now she lives in a studio apartment.

"I'd like to have the grandchildren over for the holidays, but I can't cook for so many any more. Look, it's my fingers, the arthritis."

When her husband was alive the house would smell of freshly baked challah and the floors were scrubbed to an incredible cleanliness. The table was set with the lace cloth which had come with her dowry, and the silver kiddush cup they had brought from Europe.

"My Sarah wants me to come visit with her in St. Louis over the holidays, but it's usually so hot there this time of the year. Besides, I'm afraid of the airplane, and mine back hurts and mine legs are weak."

They would like so to host the holiday meals, to bake the Challah, to prepare the matzo balls and the gefilte fish, to roast the brisket and mix the tzimmes, to make the soup and the kugel. They want to, but they can't any more. Age and infirmity simply won't permit it. And anyway the families have scattered and few want enough to bring themselves back together again. Time has passed by these bubbehs of the studio apartments (if they are lucky) and of the nursing homes (if they are not). But their fright and their loneliness remain.

"It's a 'paint' in mine back and I get weak in mine legs." And, as has been observed, although one mother can raise ten children, sometimes ten children can't take care of one mother.

I will put her in the hospital over the holidays. I will see her every day and we will talk Yiddish. Her guilt will be relieved. This will be her treatment and her cure. For surely, after the holidays have passed and she is no longer expected (by others, by herself) to do what she cannot, she will undergo a spontaneous and miraculous recovery.

She deserves it, and besides, we must protect our proud heritage.

✡

Patients/Patience

L ike Alice said, "Things get curiouser and curiouser ..." Patients. Just last week I saw on separate days elderly twin sisters, one a spinster, the other widowed, who claimed different ages. Although the medical literature has noted some delay in the birth of the second twin, five years is a bit much, wouldn't you agree? And listen to this: "Let me tell you how I hurt myself," she begins. "Well, there was this sale at Osco Drugs, and I went there with my girlfriend. I'd made a purchase, nothing big, just a few drugstore items, cosmetics and the like. They were on sale, you see. It was a year-end sale, and everything was 50 percent or more off. Anyway, I was holding the bag with the things I bought. I'd paid for them and was taking the escalator down to the basement salesroom to see if there was anything in the Kitchenware Department that I could use. My girlfriend was ahead of me on the escalator. It wasn't slippery or anything, just crowded. I was, however, wearing rubber boots because the weather man on the morning news had predicted a 70 percent possibility of snow, but it hadn't started snowing yet. Anyway, like I said, I was coming down the escalator ... now, where was I? ... Oh, yes ... like I said, I was coming down the escalator ..."

Patience with patients, like I said.

Good-bye Now

"I'm calling you during recess, Doctor, I haven't much time to talk. Just be patient and hear me out, please. I feel a little better, but I still have the pain in my hips and legs. It's worse when I write assignments on the blackboard and particularly bad when I stoop to help the kids on and off with their coats and overshoes. I tried to follow your instructions and think I did pretty well. But you've known me a long time, and even though I'm 55, I like to keep active. Not that a first-grade teacher doesn't have to be on her toes all the time, and sometimes literally! But when you live alone, it's easy just to sit around and let yourself go to pot. Which brings me to my question.

It's about the class in belly dancing I'm taking at the YWCA. I really enjoy it and would hate to have to give it up. I kind of restrain myself during the class and don't go through all the bumps and rolls, but I really get a kick out of what I do. In a strange way, it's emotionally satisfying to me; so I think it must be good exercise. I don't know exactly how to explain it. I hope, with your permission, I can keep it up.

Oh, there goes the bell, I'll have to rush back to class now. I'll call again next recess and I'll do the listening while you do the talking. Good-bye now, have to run ..."

What About

"I have this short list of questions I've written down. It won't take but a minute."

The French have a name for it, "le malade avec le petit papier" (the patient with the little paper) and she suffered the malady in both its acute and chronic forms.

"I suppose you think these are foolish questions?"

Tiny, mole-like, a 68-year-old ex-high school teacher, and a spinster.

"I saw this television program last night, 'Mucus Welaby,' or something like that. It was all about leukemia. One of the symptoms was fatigue. I often get tired. Do you think I have leukemia?"

"No, I don't think you have leukemia. I think your fatigue is natural for your age."

"Well, that's certainly a relief. Now, how about exercise? Do you think I get enough exercise?"

"As I told you last visit, you should try to walk at least a mile each day. That should be enough."

"But, should I walk the mile all at one time or can I do it in two trips; say half a mile in the morning and half a mile in the afternoon?"

"Whatever is convenient for you."

"What about sleep. Do you think eight hours is enough?"

"Are you tired when you get up in the morning?"

"No."

"Then it's sufficient."

"How about housework? Can I do my own?"

"As I've told you many times, you can do whatever you feel capable of doing."

"But what if I get tired?"

"Then you can stop and rest."

"I'm sorry to be such a bother. I'll bet you think these are stupid questions."

"There are no stupid questions, Miss Blonsky, only stupid answers."

"Then I'll continue. Now, how about ..."

◈

So, How Do I Feel?

"What happened to me?"

"You injured your shoulder."

"Is it a fracture or just a break?"

"It's just a break."

"Thank God!"

Even the equipment detail men come on as unreal if you forget for a minute what they're talking about. The other day, a salesman was trying to interest me in the latest artificial vascular grafts. "We're featuring dacron, not nylon, this season, Doctor. They come in a wide variety of sizes, and you have your choice of either woven or knitted." For a minute I thought I was buying shirts.

Speaking of clothes, you have to wear many hats in this business, and sometimes several collars. "A man for all lesions," as my old professor used to say. For instance, what would you say to the patient who histrionically claims, "I fainted dead away, completely lost my conscience. I was totally coma-toes. I'm so nervous, can't you give me a little twinkle-izer?" or how about, "I fell down and landed on my elbum. They admitted me through the emergency room, where I was x-rated. Well, that got better, but now I've got an inflation of the knee. My calf is swollen, and I can't walk. The paints are all the way into the fingers of the left foot. My son, Sherman the pharmacist, looked at it and thinks it's a rupture of the plantation muscle, not a fraction. I've been walking on stretchers since yesterday, and I'm worried because I've already got hardening of arters and varigo veins. What do you think, Doc? Am I dangerous?"

Or take your pick of the following: "My husband's a paintner, but now he schleps. He mislocated his shoulder. It got icy (frozen?), and now he's got calcimine there. I'm so relieved, I had a mimiogram x-ray of my busted and I'm negative."

Patients, they come in all varieties. The pitifully weak dystrophic who could only move by crawling in a crouch and was happy to do so; the beautiful, young model returning to college to become a teacher after her leg was amputated in a motorcycle accident; the self-indulgent teeny-bopper, complaining that the hairline-thin scar on her left hip was not tanning the same shade as the rest of her. Gypsies who pay with sweaty dollars, pulled from between pendulous breasts. The blind man who operates a newspaper and candy stand in the stock exchange and who married the severely deformed arthritic. Two old maid sisters, aging together, dying together, "Now Edna, tell the doctor where is hurts." The policeman who carefully unstraps his "38" and lays it on the table before being examined (it makes me nervous to see it there).

They are like pieces of a jigsaw puzzle, some grossly different, and many, though grossly alike, critically different. The last piece of the puzzle is, of course, the doctor himself. Just where and how he fits in makes the picture complete. In the practice of clinical medicine, where a thousand concerns clutter up a busy office afternoon, it is sometimes impossible to fit oneself exactly to each patient's particular needs. But in the attempt is the accomplishment. Maybe that's what it means when they say, "Physician, heal thyself."

Finally, the trade craft of medicine requires a sense of humor. So, when in doubt, mumble. That way you won't be thrown by all your patients with the NTB-NTG syndrome ("How do you feel today, Mr. Frankel?" "Not too bad, not too good, Doctor, but that's up to you to tell. After all, that's what I'm paying you for. So, how do I feel?").

Is there a doctor in the house?

HEALTH

※※※

The root for the word "health" is the same as that for the words "heal," "hale," and "hardy." To be dis-eased is no longer to be at ease, no longer to be "whole" (same root as "health"). But, disease is one thing, illness another. Disease is pathology, that which affects the tissues. Illness involves the psyche as well as the soma. Illness affects the persona.

To one who would treat illness, words — both listened to and spoken — are often as powerful as are drugs or instruments. Words can soothe as well as any balm, and cut as deep as any scalpel. Words, ill used, can also leave scars. The patient offers himself, and the true physician, forgetting himself as the doer, leaves a relationship and enters a process. He can thereby create a cure by linking the potentials within his patient with the possibilities within himself. To do this well, he must trust the body to exercise the capacity to heal itself. His role is merely to assist it to do so. His most valuable instrument in this process is awareness of himself. To quote Goethe, "If you would know others, study yourself, and if you would know yourself, study others." So, how does a doctor come to know himself? Why, through his patients, of course, how else?

Cost Analysis

"I'd like to give an injection of cortisone into your knee, Mr. Silver. I think it will help your arthritis."

"What will it cost me, Doctor?"

"Money should not be a consideration in making this kind of a decision, Mr. Silver, but I know you're not a rich man and I'll charge you only half of my usual fee."

"So, what will it cost me, Doctor?"

"How about $15.00, Mr. Silver?"

"How long will it take you to give the injection, Doctor?"

"Less than a minute, Mr. Silver."

"You mean, Doctor, you get $15.00 for less than a minute's work?"

"I'll tell you what, Mr. Silver, if it will make you happier, I'll leave the needle in longer."

Cindy

"Oh, Doc, you're D-y-n-a-m-i-t-e!"

"Thanks, Cindy, I get a bang out of you, too."

"But, you're not fooling now, you really mean I can go home tomorrow? Yipee! When can I have my friends over? Get off my crutches and dance again? When can I drive? Do I have to take gym? And how about ..."

"Down, girl, down, everything in due time. First we have to get you and this drugstore moved out. You've got enough cosmetics here to set up a beauty parlor."

"Aw, Doc, just because I fell off a horse and broke my leg doesn't mean I can't be well-groomed. Was that a pun? So, what's a little eye shadow, mascara and pancake makeup between us friends?"

Oh, to be a sixteen year old J.A.P. and fall off a horse into the arms of loving and indulging parents! Oh, to suffer exquisitely from youth!

"And besides, how can I stay in the running when all I can do is hop, if I can't use the war paint to get them to look twice." ("Them" being every high school jock within a five mile radius of her suburban palace.)

"Now, you listen to me, Gidget Greenblat. Narcissism is nice, but I'd like to see just a little enlightened self-interest. You do as I say, and you'll be dancing soon enough. But for the time being, I want you off your feet with that leg elevated. Understand?"

"Yes, Suh Captain, jus' like yo all say!"

"Now, Cindy, don't be a smart ass!"

"Oh, Doc, you're D-y-n-a-m-i-t-e!"

Questions and Answers

"Hello, Doctor?"

"Hello, who's this?"

"Mr. Zimmerman, Doctor."

"Yes, Mr. Zimmerman, how can I help you?"

"Well, you have my mother in the hospital and I'm calling to see how she's doing."

"She's getting along as well as can be expected, Mr. Zimmerman."

"What do you think is wrong with her, Doctor?"

"There are several possibilities, Mr. Zimmerman. I haven't quite decided as yet."

"When will you know?"

"As soon as I finish her present series of tests."

"What have the tests shown so far?"

"What we expected, Mr. Zimmerman."

"What new tests are you planning to run?"

"Some that will give us a more definite diagnosis."

"Is she getting any treatment now?"

"We're treating her symptoms. We're keeping her comfortable."

"Does she complain a great deal?"

"Not very much."

"When do you think she'll be able to come home?"

"As soon as she's well enough, Mr. Zimmerman."

"Well, thanks, Doctor, I feel better since talking to you."

"That's all right, Mr. Zimmerman, call any time."

Time

They are old, so very, very aged, and they keep growing older.

"But Doctor, why am I in pain?"

"It's simply the aging process. Not a disease, you understand, just a physiological decline. You might call it gray hair of the joints."

"But Doctor, what can I do about it?"

"Aspirin, heat, rest, not much else. It's the price you pay for senior citizenry."

"But Doctor, I didn't have the pain and stiffness last week. I never felt like this before, why now?"

The nonacceptance of aging. The bewilderment at how quickly it happened. The endless questioning. The routine visits from month to month. Prescribing enough aspirin to reach the moon, advising sufficient hot baths to fill an ocean, recommending rest enough to take a lifetime.

Moving from examining room to examining room all afternoon, like touring a museum of what has become. Attempting to stimulate interest, going on automatic pilot, feeling guilty, trying to arouse interest again.

Wouldn't it somehow be better if we were born old and infirm, with the prospect of health in the future, bringing to bear on the frivolity of youth the already accomplished intelligence of age, finally to die as old born babies, fat, healthy, pink, gurgling and wise?

I'm Not a Complainer

"Doctor, I'm not a complainer!"

Her interview and examination were accompanied by a variety of histrionic facial contortions.

"Doctor, I'm not a complainer!"

She had been hospitalized twice. Every conceivable test was negative. There were no significant physical findings. Her symptoms were vague and fit no recognized clinical pattern. When one complaint was worn out, she would quickly find another. She didn't respond to any of a variety of medications.

"Doctor, I'm not a complainer!"

Fifty-two years old, husband recently recovering from his second heart attack, one child married, the other away at college.

"Doctor, I'm not a complainer!"

No career.

No particular hobbies, avocational or recreational interests.

No intimate circle of friends.

"Doctor, I'm not a complainer!"

No strong religious affiliation.

No close family ties.

No organic pathology.

"Doctor, I'm not a complainer!"

※

How's Her Appetite?

I said, "How's her appetite? Is she getting enough to eat?"

He said, "I think so, Doctor. Of course, I soften all her food. But she even has a hard time handling mashed things. She can't hardly swallow anything but liquids now."

She didn't say anything. She couldn't. She just started to weep.

I said, "There, there, don't cry. It'll be all right" (which was a lie).

He said, "She's having more trouble breathing now. She sometimes gasps."

I said, "You must see that she uses the oxygen mask when this happens. It's not an uncommon occurrence in patients with her disease."

She was sobbing harder and harder, and her head fell to one side and she started to drool. He carefully folded a white handkerchief under her chin to catch the spittle.

Then he said, "I think she needs something to support her head now, Doctor. She's so weak that it keeps falling backwards when she sits in the wheelchair."

And I said, "I can see she's getting weaker. I'll prescribe a collar to help support her head."

And all the while she wept, the tears running down her cheeks to mix with the saliva running into the handkerchief.

Then he said, "When shall I bring her back to see you again, Doctor?"

And I thought of saying, "There's no need to bring her back again. She's not going to live very long now. It's best you take her home and as gently as possible prepare for her death."

But I didn't say that.

Because I couldn't say that.

And besides, they both already knew it.

◼

No Problem at All

As soon as I walked into the examining room, I could smell her bad teeth.

"I got it in a fight with my boyfriend. He came at me with a broken coke bottle."

The emergency room had done a good job. She had about fifty stitches, but the fine scar would balance the one on the opposite cheek.

"Where is your boyfriend now?"

"Freddie? He's at home. He's really not a bad sort. Just gets a little rambunctious when he's drunk.

"Does he attack you often?"

"Like I said, just when he's drunk."

"You must love him to put up with it."

"Love him, hell! He keeps me supplied," as she thrusts her scar-tracked arms toward me.

"I can see that you get to a methadone clinic. I think you ought to give it a try. Heroin is a bad one-way street."

"No use. I've already tried to kick it, twice. I just can't do it."

"Well, let me send you upstairs to the lab for a hemoglobin. You must have had a significant loss of blood with that facial laceration. We can talk about the heroin problem when you come back down. But I don't know how they're going to draw blood from those arms."

"Don't worry, Doc. Just tell them to give me the syringe. I'll get the blood for them. It's no problem at all."

The Number Game

"Nu! So what was the number of my cholesterol this time?"

"It was normal, Mrs. Ginsburg."

"Of course it was normal, Doctor, but what was the number?"

"Isn't it enough to know it was normal, Mrs. Ginsburg? Why do you have to know the specific value?"

"My friend, Sylvia Cohen, who sees Dr. Weiss told me he told her that her number was 175. Was mine higher or lower than that?"

"Yours was 190. Does that make you feel good or bad?"

"I'm no dummy, Doctor. In this case, it isn't the higher the better, but I don't mind being higher than Sylvia, just so long as it is normal. Now, how about the sugar?"

"110."

"Last time is was 100."

I assure you, Mrs. Ginsburg, there is nothing to worry about."

"And the blood?"

"RBC 5.1, hemoglobin 15, hematocrit 44, WBC 8.3, differential within normal limits, and sed rate 21."

"You're confusing me, Doctor."

"I mean to, Mrs. Ginsburg."

"Now you're teasing me, Doctor."

"I also mean to do that, Mrs. Ginsburg."

"If you were to add all those numbers together, would it mean anything, Doctor?"

"It would, indeed, Mrs. Ginsburg. It would mean that I didn't know anything about the practice of medicine."

"Maybe you could discover a new test."

"You have all the values now, Mrs. Ginsburg. Why don't you try it? You just add them all together and divide by your age. You can compare your result with your friend Sylvia's."

"That sounds like a good idea, Doctor. I'll let you know as soon as I figure it out."

"Tell you what, Mrs. Ginsburg, don't call me with the results. Call Dr. Weiss."

Lues

The Italians called it the French disease. The French called it the Italian disease. We call it syphilis, and you can't get it from a dirty toilet seat.

"But I swear I haven't had intercourse with anyone but my wife!"

A middle-aged executive, understandably distraught with his diagnosis.

I don't know what to say, so I say nothing. I just sit there.

"But, Doctor, I swear I haven't had intercourse with anyone but ... my wife?"

It was immortalized by the Italian physician-poet, Girolamo Fracastoro, in his poem, "Syphilis sive morbus gallicus," first published in 1530, in which he described the plight of a shepherd smitten with the disease for blaspheming the sun god. The word "syphilis" itself derives from the Greek and means "shameful, hideous, repulsive."

"And remember, men, you can't tell the clean ones from the dirty ones by the way they look."

Basic training VD lecture.

"Always visit a pro station after you've had a piece, and turn up for short arm inspection every Friday."

I had nightmares for a week after the horror movie they showed us.

"Don't forget, it's a court-martial if you come down with a case of VD."

We used to joke about it ("Did you hear about the patient who flunked his Wassermann Test?"). But it's not funny. It can affect seriously almost every organ system of the body. It is so protean it has been called the "great imitator." It was once said that if you understood syphilis, you understood half of medicine.

"Have you ever had 'bad blood'?" An elderly black man is the patient.

"No, Suh, but I once had a 'haircut' (chancre) on my privates."

Originally, it was treated by serial injections of heavy metal. They used to say, "One night with Venus, a lifetime with Mercury." Occasionally, such heavy metal deposits reveal themselves on an x-ray of an elderly society matron presenting herself for an unrelated condition. "To ask or not to ask," that is always the question. The doctor should know, but the patient must be assured of his discretion.

"You've never had a series of injections for an infectious disease, have you?"

"Not that I recall."

"Perhaps when you were younger, try to remember now. Were you ever treated for a venereal infection?"

"Not that I remember."

This doesn't say no and, no doubt, she doesn't recall. She doesn't want to. I don't press it. A few simple tests will tell me if she is cured. If not, we can treat her.

Columbus' crew was reputed to have brought it to Europe from the new world during one of his many voyages, and the worst news is that it seems like it's coming back. Penicillin had it by the throat for awhile, but resistant strains of treponema (the causative organism) have developed and, in some places, syphilis is reaching near epidemic proportions.

Many famous people, both notable and notorious, have had the disease. The famous English anatomist surgeon, John

Hunter, inoculated himself with a discharge from an infected patient to prove it was different than gonorrhea. The patient, however, had both, Hunter got both, and for awhile the profession thought they were the same disease. On a more notorious note, the Chicago gangster, Al Capone, carried his syphilis to the grave.

French, Italian, or Spanish — it looks like syphilis may be around in one guise or another as long as people are, and as long as they act like people should or shouldn't. Well, at least you can't get it from a dirty toilet seat.

More Time

It's never easy to accept, no matter how many times it happens, no matter how often you see it. And there it is again, blinking into life on the x-ray viewbox. That ominous sunburst of bone, startling in its contrast to the delicate tracery of the normal shaft of her youthful femur, terrible in its promise of almost certain death. Despite amputation, radiation, chemotherapy. Despite anything and everything.

Now the parent is looking at you. The parent wants to know. The parent deserves to know.

"Jennifer is only ten, Mrs. Clark. We are going to have to disarticulate her hip. She will require cobalt radiation treatments. We'll pump her full of chemotoxic agents. In spite of all this, she will probably die within a year."

"Please, Doctor, she's such a wonderful child. The joy of the family. She planned to be a dancer. Please, Doctor, say she'll be well!"

"I can't say that, Mrs. Clark. I wish I could, but I simply can't."

What kind of nonsense is this, can such a thing ever really be so?

"I was just joking, Mr. Levy. You must forgive my black sense of humor. The pressures of my practice and all. Just a playful prank. A jest, no more. Excuse me for making sport of you. It's nothing, nothing, I assure you. Just the sun rising behind the x-ray viewbox. The films are negative. Everything's normal. Do you hear? Everything is perfectly normal. There is nothing to worry about."

And to the child (why are they always the most beautiful ones?): "Now, Tommy, you run home and play. Here, buy yourself an ice cream soda on the way."

You check the name on the film again. Maybe there's been a mistake. No, It's her film, Rachel Smith, plain as day. The parents are waiting. The father speaks.

"Is there a cure, Doctor?"

You want so to weave fantasy with hope: "Certainly, Mr. Black. There is a cure. I have it here in my hand. A single magic pill. A secret balm. A painless injection. Take Beverly home now, let her get a good night's rest, and by tomorrow morning ..."

But you say instead: "We find something here a little more serious than what we had originally expected."

Why do we always use the first person plural when we're talking about a malignancy? How about a little first person singular honesty?

"Like I said, Mr. Grady, Harold will have to lose a leg. But don't worry, we'll fit him with a nice new one, almost as good as a natural limb. You have no idea how advanced prosthetic technology is. What with plastic and suction sockets, we'll have him back hopping in no time."

"That's wonderful; we'll be able to take our Florida vacation after all. Did you hear that, Harold? You won't have to miss the Cub Scout meeting next month. Doctor says everything is going to be all right. Did you hear that, son? Everything's going to be all right!"

It's always easier to break the news on familiar turf, in the home park, so to speak: "It'll be necessary to hospitalize Robert for further tests and examinations."

There are two schools of thought concerning letting the parents and the child know. The tell-it-to-them-all-at-once school and the let-it-sink-in-slowly school. Needless to say, the latter is the more popular: "Do I know what's wrong? Not exactly. There are a few conditions I suspect. I'll know more after I have the test results. Then we can talk about it."

Finally, this guide for the perplexed offers the following variations on the theme, "Death be not proud" and other assorted TV bullshit: "Nonetheless, though, you mustn't lose hope."

"A major medical breakthrough may occur at any time."

"I'd like to get another opinion."

"Let me review the examinations more thoroughly before reaching a diagnosis. I require more time."

Yes, That's it. More time. I simply require more time.

Instructions

"Bathe it three times a day in warm water. Elevate it on two pillows higher than your heart. Massage it with rubbing alcohol or cold cream, always remembering to massage toward, never away, from the heart. Apply ice either in an ice bag or a plastic sack. Hold it in a sling. Take two aspirins for pain every three to four hours. Rest it as much as you can. Apply dry heat. Apply moist heat. Don't do any overhead work and don't lift anything that weighs more than five pounds, remembering always to lift close to your body. Perform all routine tasks at eye or waist level. Use a firm bed and straight-back chairs. Bend from the knees, not from the back. Apply heat nightly. Apply cold regularly. Have your pharmacist get in touch with me for a prescription. Let me know when you would like the surgery scheduled. Here is my nurse. She'll make an appointment. Exercise it regularly as instructed. Stay off of it. Use it. Rest it. Exercise it. Elevate it. Lower it. Heat it. Cool it.

Check with me in the morning. Don't call me. Call me. Don't call me. Call me, call me, call me ..."

Me

"**W**hy did you try to fool the nurses by heating the thermometer, so it would look like you were running a fever?"

"I wanted to stay in the hospital."

"But look at the trouble you caused us. Here, we've all been trying to find out what's wrong, running all sorts of tests, worrying about your diagnosis."

"I wanted to stay in the hospital. I wanted somebody to worry about me, not just my diagnosis."

"But we wanted you to get well, to go back to your home, to be able to take care of your husband and children."

"I wanted to stay in the hospital. I wanted someone to take care of me."

"It was a foolish thing to do. You should have realized that sooner or later someone would discover that you were faking the fever."

"I wanted to stay in the hospital. I wanted somebody to worry about me. I wanted someone to take care of me. I wanted somebody to discover *me*!"

I'm Worried

"**I**'m worried."

"No need to worry, there's less than a one percent chance."

"But if it's me, then it's 100%."

"I'm just running the test to be absolutely certain. I really don't think you have it."

"But you looked concerned when you suggested further x-rays and a bone scan."

"I'm always concerned, but that doesn't mean that I'm worried."

"And your associate didn't say a word when he examined me. Besides, he frowned when he read my record?"

"Would you like to read your record?"

"No, it would just confuse me, and I would worry more."

"Honestly, I don't think you have anything to fear."

"I trust you, you know that."

"I appreciate your trust."

"Nonetheless, I'm worried!"

PAIN

I speak of pain. Pain, the ancient Greeks equated it with punishment, penalty, payment; hence the word. Pain, housed in the thalamus, the "inner room," the most primitive chamber of the brain. Pain, which sweeps the spectrum from uneasiness through discomfort to agony, evoking at best the wish to avoid and at worst the desperation to escape. Pain, the inevitable expression of excess of any pleasure. Pain, the protector; pain, the leveler; pain, the common human denominator. The way we know ourselves, through pain.

Albert Schweizer regarded it the true brotherhood of man, "The fellowship of those who bear the mark of pain." Yet, it is not together that we feel pain, for by its nature it is a solitary experience. Pain, the final unmasking, and in this nakedness, its cruelest shame. Is then the knowledge that someone who understands this is at your side its most powerful anodyne? I do think so.

It has been truly said that if a doctor has not felt pain, his education is sadly incomplete.

Gout

It's no joke (cartoons of a gluttonous aristocrat, his face contorted in pain, his swollen foot elevated on several pillows, to the contrary), and it is small consolation that historically it has afflicted such wise and famous men as Henry VIII, Kubla Kahn, Luther, Goethe, Charlemagne, Milton, Cromwell, Isaac Newton, Galileo, Charles Darwin, Theodore Roosevelt, and William Pitt the Elder, to mention but a few.

I speak of gout, the ancient disease once called the "Rheumatism of the rich" and now known to be a metabolic flaw, which is not caused, only aggravated, by overindulgence in food or drink.

The word "Gout" originated from the Latin "Gutta," a drop, as the inflammation was supposedly due to the discharge, drop-by-drop, of harmful humors into the joints. Specifically, gout is caused by either too much production or too little excretion of the metabolite, uric acid. With its accumulation in or around the affected part, usually a joint, attacks can be triggered by stress, gastronomic, physical or emotional.

Gout plays no national favorites, even though the French claim they have goût for the taste, while the English have gout for the result. However, it does show a strong sexual predilection, 95% of gout sufferers being males who are intensely achievement-oriented. This striking correlation between gout and prominence (it has been shown statistically that men with high I.Q.'s and increased blood uric acid levels are more likely to be leaders) has never been adequately explained.

Gout is an ancient disease described in the Bible, "And Esau in the thirty and ninth year of his reign was diseased in his feet, until his disease was exceedingly great: yet in his disease he sought not the Lord, but to the physician ..." (II Chronicles 16:12). In fact, Aaron's admonition to his sons that they not partake of wine, "Else they die," may indeed refer to the association of severe attacks of gout with alcoholic intake.

Gout was not only believed due to high living — a Spanish proverb says: "Gout is cured by walling up the mouth" — but also lechery. Benjamin Franklin, another notable gout sufferer, wrote, "Be temperate in wine, in eating, girls, and sloth, or the gout will seize you and plague you both" (*Poor Richard's Almanac,* 1734). The father of medicine, Hippocrates, in his aphorisms, states, "Eunuchs do not take the gout, nor become bald ... a young man does not take the gout until he indulges in coition." Though overstated, there seems to be a measure of truth in these observations, as the process of gouty inflammation occurs only in the presence of male hormones.

Though it can affect any joint, gout usually begins in the great toe. This involvement is called podagra, literally, "a foot attack." "Full soon the sad effect of this (port wine)/his frame began to show/for that old enemy the gout/had taken him in toe." (Thomas Hood, 1799-1845). The pain is almost unbearable and has been eloquently described by many great authors, including Jonathan Swift, "Dear, honest Ned is in the gout/lies racked with pain, and you without./How patiently you hear him groan!/ How glad the case is not your own!"

Modern treatment consists of reasonable living habits, including proper diet and exercise (overweight, and too little or even too much exercise with diminished fluid intake can trigger an episode of gout), and, for the acute attack, colchicine, a drug known to the ancients as both a specific for easing the pain of gout and an assassin's poison, causing violent diarrhea and death. Attacks can be prevented by drugs which either limit the production of uric acid or encourage its excretion.

Well, with all the folklore, it is sometimes difficult to sort out fact from fiction, but venery and overeating apart, gout is very real to those who suffer it. Real, and no joking matter!

❖

Sun Pictures

His mind was supersaturated with latent images. They were like the sun pictures he used to develop when he was a child. By exposing to the sun a specially treated paper in contact with a negative, a clear photograph would slowly develop. In the same fashion, forgotten but never lost moments in his past were clarified intensely when exposed to enough light.

"It's not that it hurts so much. It's just that it looks so awful, and I can't fit into petite shoes any longer."

Her name was Fannie Caplan. Everything about her was grotesquely artificial, from her tinted hair and false eyelashes to her carefully cosmetized legs. Even her name was phony. She spelled it Fanye Kaplawn. She was complaining about her feet.

"I really wish you could do something about them." Heels are getting higher this year and toes will be more pointed. I don't know how I'm going to wear the new shoe styles."

He had to answer her. She was, after all, his patient, and he had a moral, as well as a contractual obligation to answer her questions. But she was only fifty years old, and he always had difficulty with this kind of truth.

"You see," he began, "the diabetes has progressed to the point where the circulation to the legs has been compromised. It is in fact so poor that the tissues can no longer survive. The question is not whether or not we should take off the leg, but rather at what level should we amputate."

"I help my husband every day. I don't think he can run the grocery without me. He has a bad back, you know."

"I will do my very best. I'll save as much of your leg as I can."

"Those crazy designers. There ought to be a law. They just change styles in order to sell more shoes. It's the same thing every year. Throw away a whole closet full just because the style changed."

"I understand how you feel, but I'll have you back walking within a month, new leg and all."

"How about the other one? Just look at those feet. Did you ever see such bad corns in your life?"

"I'll do my best. I promise, I swear, I affirm I'll do my best!"

Why do things get so mixed up? Or is it that they are not mixed up; they are just the same and he never recognized it before? Just like the sun pictures. All you need is enough light to see what's on the magic paper.

Never Again

When you're a balding, overweight, diabetic Jewish bachelor and you've worked all your life as a butcher in partnership with your brother-in-law, you really don't have much going for you, particularly if you're about to have a leg amputated.

"I won't let you do it ... I'd rather die!"

I held the trump card. I knew that sooner or later he'd find there was no alternative. I tried to be supportive without intruding. I let him mourn the loss of his limb, permitting him to come to this realization in his own time and way. He clutched my hand as he cried his 65-year-old tears.

"Will I walk again," he sobbed.

"Yes, you will walk again."

"And drive a car, and play golf?"

"Yes, and drive a car and play golf."

"But I'll never be able to go into the meat freezer again."

The meat freezer.

Never again.

The meat freezer.

Never ... never again.

Maybe It's the IUD

"**A**nd besides that, I've got pains in my arms, shoulders, back of the neck, in my hips, knees, ankles and feet."

She was heavy, but not fat. She had a poor complexion. She looked weary, bored, and at least ten years older than her stated age of 27.

"Did you injure yourself?"

"No, not that I can remember. Do you think it's the chair I use at work? I sometimes have to sit at a typewriter for three to four hours straight."

"That may be part of the cause. Have you had any fever or chills?"

"No. I haven't been ill recently. Maybe it's because I've been on a diet."

"Perhaps. Do you get any regular exercise?"

"Not much. Just walk to the train in the morning and hang on a strap all the way to work. Repeat the same act at night on the way back."

"What hurts the most today?"

"Today it's mostly my back. Sometimes the top and sometimes the lower part. Sometimes all over."

"Can you take off work for a few days, stay in bed, put heat on your back, just rest."

"It's not possible. I need the money. I can't take the time off. Besides, I live by myself in an efficiency and there's no one to help me there.

"How about your parents or friends? Isn't there someone who could give you a hand?"

"I don't see my mother much since she remarried. I don't want to ask her for help. I keep pretty much to myself. I don't have many close friends, just a lot of acquaintances. Isn't there a shot or something you could give me?"

"I think you need more than just a shot."

"I use an intra-uterine device. Perhaps that's what's causing the trouble. Do you think it could be? Maybe it's the IUD?
Maybe it's the IUD?"

※

My Child Never Cried

My child never cried. He was a six-year-old black boy. You
couldn't really tell how beautiful he was because he was
burned over 50% of his body, including parts of his face, but
you sensed it anyway. His life was sustained by intravenous
feedings, and because of his age, the extent of skin loss secondary to burn, and the size of his veins, he required a
"cutdown" for their administration.

This minor surgical procedure, in which a vein is located
under local anesthesia through a small incision and a cannula
inserted therein, had to be repeated frequently because either
the cannula would pull out of the vein or it would clog up because his fragile tissues could not support the apparatus.
Cutdowns were performed at the bedside by the intern assigned
to the Children's Burn Service. That was me.

It was the fourth cutdown I was doing on him, and he never
cried. It was unnerving. He didn't make a sound. He lay there
immobile, his flesh stinking with burn, and he stared at me
with hot eyes, black as smoke, from behind his heavily ban-
daged body, his tiny lips firmly closed, paling in clenched
tension. It was a frustrating job. To change a cutdown at 3 A.M.
after a 12-hour day on the wards was a drag of the first order.
It was the middle of July, and County Hospital wasn't air con-
ditioned. It was muggy; sweat dripped into my eyes, and I was
having a hard time finding the vein. My mouth tasted sleep. A
small lamp lit the bedside area at which I was working. The
rest of the stuffy room was dark. I had been at the job for over
ten minutes, and as I probed through the bleeding tissues, seek-
ing the tiny vessel, I could hear turnings and whimperings from

the other 30-odd restless children in the ward, moving painfully through their burned-out dreams. But my child never cried.

I injected more novocaine. I could never tell whether or not he really needed it. He never talked. He just stared at me with an awful mixture of trust and hate. And he never cried. So, I injected more novocaine. I kept searching for the vein. I would find it if it took all night. The wound was like a mouth. A blistered mouth that mocked me as I struggled to find the vein. I would find the vein and place the cannula, and then I would again pour life into him. We all knew he would die, as indeed he must also have known. Children with over 50% third degree body burns seldom live. And as I bent over his tiny, charred body in the middle of that hot, dark night, alone on that restless ward in that lonely building, I realized I was not searching only for his vein, but also for something within myself. I was trying not only to save his life, but something in my own as well.

My child never cried. Later perhaps I would. For both of us.

I'll Wait

A seventy-year-old woman.
"It hurts all over, there isn't a place it doesn't pain."

She suffered all the infirmities of her age, including advanced degenerative arthritis in all her joints.

"Where does it hurt today, Mrs. Goldstein?"

"It hurts every place, and with my Max gone, all I want to do is die."

"Don't talk that way, Mrs. Goldstein. You still have a lovely family left."

"Some lovely family. Sadie lives in Miami Beach and Ruth and her fancy lawyer husband live in New York City. I get cards from the grandchildren on Mother's Day and flowers by wire on my birthday."

The same complaint. It never changes. Only the face, only the voice changes.

"In the last year two of my closest friends passed on. Everything hurts, Doctor. I think my Max is getting lonesome for me."

"You'll be better, Mrs. Goldstein. I'll give you some new medicine that'll make you feel better."

"I hope it helps, Doctor, but I doubt it will."

"You'll feel better, Mrs. Goldstein. Just wait. You'll see."

"I'll wait, Doctor. That's about all I can do. I'll wait."

Please Explain It to Her

Everything about her seemed so fragile, from her soft white hair to her heavily veined hands; as if she could be blown apart by a mere puff of wind. Everything, that is, except the eyes. They were wide and bright and still darted about curiously as she perched on her wheelchair like some fragile bird about to take wing.

I spoke to the accompanying son.

"She ought to be fine now. Her latest x-ray shows that the wrist fracture is healed. All she needs is some local heat, massage and plenty of exercise. I'll send a physical therapy prescription on to the nursing home."

"I don't want to go back to the nursing home." She's suddenly aware and alive, peeking at her son through the uriniferous veil which surrounds her."

"I don't want to go back. I want to come home with you."

"But, Mother, we all decided that Twin-Oaks Manor was, all things considered, the best place for you to stay."

"Nothing considered! No one asked me what I felt was best. I'm tired of living out of a single drawer with some nurse telling me when to eat and when to sleep, and no privacy at all."

"But, Mother, Gertrude and I thought you'd be happier away from the noise and confusion of the children."

"Noise and confusion, nonsense. Have you ever been in a nursing home during tray serving time?"

"But, Mother, if you don't like Twin-Oaks, we can always look for a more suitable place."

"As far as you're concerned, the most suitable place for me would be in a wooden box lying next to your father. All right, if that's what you want, I'll go back to that damned hole — I'll go back there and die!"

"But, Mother, be reasonable. Doctor, explain it to her. Won't you please explain it to her?"

The Painting

He was sensitive, a dreamer, an artist. While sketching by the lake, he went for a swim. He was thinking about his painting and didn't notice the speedboat. The boat was heading into the sun, and its driver failed to see him in the water. He was caught in the propellers. When they pulled him out, he was missing both legs.

"That first night was a terrible experience." He told me several days later from his bed on the Intensive Care Unit, "All I can remember now are those figures moving about as they pulled me from the water. Shapes and sizes, color, light and dark. I tried to make sense out of it and couldn't. It was like a painting, like a giant abstract painting. There were forms. There was tension and movement. The only way I could make any sense of it was to see it like a painting. You see, it wasn't real. It wasn't representational. It was like a piece of abstract art. Imagery, you know — symbolic. It was structure and balance. But it didn't tell a story — you had to bring your own meaning to it. That's the only way I could make any sense out of it. Can you understand that? Can you understand what it means to go

138

for a swim and have both your legs cut off? Can you understand why I had to make some sense of it? Can you understand?

Later that night he came to his bedside and sat. "I want to help you," he whispered, as he looked at the way the sheet dipped where the legs had been.

"How can you help me, you can't understand, so how can you help?"

"Of course, I can't understand," he whispered, "but nonetheless, I want to help."

"Help? But how?"

"First, if you'll permit me, I would like to kneel by your bedside and wash your feet."

And there in the darkness they held hands and silently wept together.

She is All the Others

"Hello, Doctor, I'm sorry to disturb you at home, but you did ask me to call."

"That's right, Mrs. Sutton, I'm glad you did. How is the new medicine working out?"

"Well, we've only been on it a few days, but Larry seems to be much better."

"I'm happy to hear that. What changes have you noticed?"

"He's less tight around the hips and knees and easier to dress. I just have the feeling that he's more relaxed, looser all over."

"Anything else?"

"Yes, he cooperates a little better when I feed him and even seems to relax more when he's bathed."

"That's wonderful, Mrs. Sutton. Have you noticed any side effects yet?"

"Nothing you cautioned me to watch for, Doctor. Oh yes, there is one thing. Every time I change his diaper, his urine seems more heavily colored. The diaper is more yellow than it used to be."

"That's not unusual with this medicine, Mrs. Sutton, I wouldn't worry about it at all. Has Larry indicated that he's feeling better since starting the drug?"

"Well, he can't talk, of course. But I sense that he's less nervous about being handled than before."

"What dose do we have him on now?"

"Two teaspoons a day, one in the morning, one in the evening."

"Good, let's keep him on that for another two weeks and then report back to me by phone, and we'll see if we have to change the dosage schedule."

"I'll do just that. Thanks much, Doctor. I'll phone you again in two weeks. Good-bye."

"Good-bye, Mrs. Sutton."

She is not, however, the usual overanxious mother. And Larry is not the average sick child. He is a 26-year-old brain-damaged cerebral spastic who has been retarded from birth. He has never walked, crawled, sat without support, or talked. He has no control over his bowel or bladder and must be managed in diapers. He cannot feed or dress himself. He requires constant attention and care and is totally dependent on others for his survival. She is all the others, and he is her entire world. For whatever purpose and to whatever end, she loves him, deeply, gently and with no remorse.

STUDENTS

❇❇❇

The premise with which you start is that everyone is potentially somebody more. This possibility is the only thing worth teaching anyone, which is all right because you can't teach anybody anything anyway; all you can do is to guide, or better yet inspire, each to teach him or herself. Most of the important things a good student needs to learn he already knows. He just has to be shown that facts can be recognized and knowledge imparted, but the synthesis of understanding lies neither in preceptorship or instruction, but rather somewhere within himself. It's there; it just has to be nurtured and coaxed out of hiding, acknowledged, learned anew.

The enemy of such "learning from the left" is boredom. Modern-day students are too sophisticated to use the term. Instead they say, "It's irrelevant." I suppose relevance is ultimately a function of context, yet when you are dealing with life and the incalculable variety of its human practitioners, everything is relevant. Another common complaint is, "That's old hat, it's not new." Well, to the curious mind, everything can be new. As the great physiologist, Claude Bernard, once observed, "Scientific discovery is seeing something that everyone has seen and thinking something that no one has thought." The student's mind should be constantly startled by these newnesses. Each instruction should be a discovery. The shock of all this sometimes hurts, but such pain is always enlightening.

Everything isn't simple; some things are very complicated. One is constantly balancing facts, trying to separate events from processes. On the other hand, there's no sense in acting like Hamlet and making a simple situation more complicated than it need be, even less than trying like Othello to simplify what is most complicated. Students have to learn these things. First, of course, teachers should know them.

One of the important things a young doctor must learn is to enlarge his humanity while pursuing his scientific vocation. Caring is the chicken soup of medical practice. It's the basic stock in the recipe for a good physician. All a patient really knows about his doctor is if he or she is thorough and if he or she is kind. However, these two traits are about ninety percent of the whole armamentarium of successful doctorhood. With them, you don't need much else working for you; without one, it's a hard trip, and without both, it's nigh impossible.

Studentry isn't a developmental phase; it's an inclination of the mind. Personally, I teach to learn. I enjoy students. I hope I'll always be one.

I Stopped Feeling Sorry Long Ago

It was early November, it was late afternoon, and it was rain-ing. I was completing the sixth month of my internship, as-signed to the Cook County Hospital Emergency Room. I enjoyed it. However, the rain had cut visibility and business both to zero. The hospital guards were even permitting some of the local indigents to escape from the cold and wet of the streets into the somber warmth of the dingy waiting room where they lay stretched out on hard wooden benches, covering them-selves with newspapers for blankets.

My change of shift was 20 minutes off. I was thumbing a text on the emergency treatment of acute poisoning while in-termittently staring through a dirty window at the dirtier street outside, pelted with waves of seemingly endless rain. Just as I was about to fix my third cup of coffee, he appeared at the door.

He was black, middle-aged, drenched to the skin and shiv-ering. Also, he was blind. You have to understand, I have this thing about blindness. A friend of mine studying to be a psy-chiatrist once told me it was an upward displacement of an unresolved castration complex. Well, maybe. Anyhow, my feel-ings about the blind have always been gut-strong. His was a familiar story. He was on welfare, living alone in a basement apartment. Borderline nutrition and the dampness of his flat led from a simple cold to a persistent cough with chills and fever. He couldn't afford public transportation. He walked to the hospital for help. By the time he arrived, he was so wet you couldn't tell the color of his clothes.

Fortunately, my examination revealed nothing beyond a severe upper respiratory infection. Certainly no pneumonia. At worst, early bronchitis. I dressed him in hospital garb, put-ting his wet clothes to dry on the radiator, gave him a cup of hot coffee, and wrote two prescriptions, one for an antibiotic, the other for cough syrup. I really wanted to hospitalize him but he wasn't that sick, and I would have been severely criticized for unnecessarily utilizing a bed. The pharmacy was due to close shortly and I didn't want him to get lost getting there, so I decided to walk over with him.

The pharmacy was indeed closed when we arrived, the service window shut, and the over-varnished door locked. I rang the emergency bell. No answer. I rang again. Still no answer. I rang once more, this time insistently. The door opened and I was confronted by an elderly man.

He was shorter than I, and what little hair he had was gray and disheveled. He badly needed a shave. He wore a short dirty hospital coat with the sleeves rolled up. It was wrinkled and stained and missing several buttons. In his right hand he held a piece of fried chicken, a bit of which he was still chewing.

"Well," he snapped, "what do you want?"

"I have a patient here with a bad respiratory infection. He needs two prescriptions filled."

"The pharmacy is closed," he replied. "He can get them filled elsewhere or come back in the morning." He started to close the door.

"But he hasn't got the money to pay for them privately, and besides, he's blind, and it's difficult for him to travel."

"I told you we're closed. I've worked all day and now I'm finished."

At this, he turned and walked toward the back of the pharmacy. I followed him through the door between shelves of bottles and jars into a room heavy with pungent medicinal odors. "Look, I'm sorry to be late." I was begging by now. "And I'm sorry I interrupted your dinner, but this poor man could really use the medicine today. It would be a mitzvah if you could take a few minutes to fill the prescriptions." I hardly expected the vigor of his response.

"Mitzvah!" he exploded. "You speak to me of good deeds! What do you call working in this crummy place day after day, having to spill out the rest of my life serving endless lines of miserable people, if not a good deed? Isn't that enough? Can't I even have my peace at the end of the day? You can feel sorry if you want. I stopped feeling sorry long ago. I tried it and it doesn't change a thing. Do you think I was always employed in a place like this? Before the Depression, I used to have a store of my own. A fancy place in a good neighborhood ... But the competition of the big chains was finally just too much. I lost everything, and here I am, in the back of a crummy county hospital pharmacy, eating a chicken dinner out of a greasy paper bag. So don't talk to me about good deeds."

We found ourselves quietly looking at each other. He had been gesticulating wildly in the air with the chicken, but his right arm now hung limp at his side. After a few minutes of silence, I turned to leave. I was almost to the door when I heard him mumble.

"Oh, what the hell, give me the prescriptions."

It didn't take long to prepare the medication. I tried to thank him as he handed them to me.

"Forget your thanks," he said. "Just leave quickly so I can finish eating and read my newspaper."

It was still raining when we walked back to the emergency room. It was also dark outside, and the unshielded light fixtures in the high ceilings cast a naked glare on the cold, cracked walls of the hollow corridors. I was caught somewhere between that bitter disillusioned man's loneliness and the ever renewing excitements of my young enthusiasm. The blind man was also in there someplace. In fact, as we walked silently along with his arm gripping mine for guidance, I had difficulty telling where his hand ended and my arm began. It suddenly seemed to me as though I would never be wholly rid of him, and I felt strangely as if I were my own father.

What Happened Next

What happened next shocked them all. The cat, after all the difficulty they had putting her under, awakened with a horrible screech, wrenched herself free of the restraining board, at the same time pulling the intravenous out and the electrodes off her head, bolted from the table and started frantically running about the room.

"God damn it, Ed, can't you keep that fuckin' feline asleep!"

The four of them on team B had not yet gathered all their data on the physiology experiment when this happened. They still had to administer three more drugs intravenously, record, observe and compare their effect on the cat's brain through the electroencephalographic tracing.

"I picked her because I thought she looked like an easy cat to anesthetize," Ed was speaking now, "but it took three of us to hold the bitch just to get her to breathe a little chloroform."

They were all chasing her. Fortunately, one of them had been quick-witted enough to close the door when the cat made her leap for freedom. She wasn't going to be taken without a fight, had scratched the first pursuer who grabbed her, and was now perched atop the dissecting table, her back arched, her eyes narrowed, and her teeth barred.

"What the hell are we going to do now? I hope my patients don't respond like this during surgery. It's enough to make you go into psychiatry or dermatology, one of the quieter specialties."

"Psychiatric patients act like this all the time, you dummy. And dermatology is a little bit too dull, even for you. The patients never get well and never die. I'd say with your background and particular skills, you're rather cut out to use a proctoscope. You know what a proctoscope is, don't you?"

"Of course I do, you idiot, it's a hollow tube with an asshole at each end!"

"All right you guys, come on now, stop jazzing around. Let's figure out how to get this damned cat back on the table, or we'll never make it to clinical conference next period."

They planned a strategy. One of them borrowed four pairs of heavy gloves from the laboratory deiner. Thus protected, they surrounded the cat and closed in, each bearing a handful of chloroform-soaked cotton.

The cornered animal struggled, scratched a bit, but was finally overcome. They carried her limp form back to the restraining board and securely strapped her down.

"She's a big one, isn't she? I wonder why she struggled so hard. We never had this trouble with a cat before."

"She sure is big. At least it'll be easier getting the IV going again. Here, give me a hand getting it restarted."

They finished the experiment, this time giving enough anesthetic to make sure the animal didn't re-awaken. Then they sacrificed her quickly by running green soap through the intravenous.

"Who wants to autopsy her?"

"It's not in the protocol this time, there's nothing to see, and besides, we'll be late for our next class."

"Still, I'd like to. It's been a long time since I've been in a cat. Ever since comparative anatomy. Yes, I'd like to. Just for kicks."

"You do what you want. Just remind me not to refer you any of my patients when you become a surgeon. You're knife-happy, you know, and that can be dangerous."

They left and he was alone with the cat. He bundled it into a towel and carried it down the corridor to the animal autopsy room. "She sure is heavy. Maybe she has a tumor or something," he thought, his excitement mounting with the prospect of an interesting dissection.

He switched on the light in the autopsy laboratory. He was alone because the experiment did not call for dissection, and the rest of his class had left for the clinical conference. He, however, never let pass the opportunity to dissect, even if it meant missing another medical school activity.

"So, I'll be a little late. I hear it's not such an interesting case today anyway," he mumbled to himself as he slipped into a dissecting gown.

He spread the animal, face up, on the perforated metal autopsy table, powdered his hands, and donning a pair of surgical gloves, he arranged a few instruments on a Mayo stand to his right. Then he cut a path through the abdominal hair with an electric razor.

Next, he placed a long midline incision through the skin of the abdomen and the underlying musculature. He enlarged the incision to the peritoneum. Dark blood was oozing from the

147

wound. This he sponged up. Then he opened the peritoneum with scissors, and spreading the edges of the incision with a heavy, self-retaining retractor, he entered the abdomen. A large organ filling the pelvic cavity pushed its way well up into his field. He opened it and could not believe what it contained. The cat was pregnant. She bore five kittens, neatly packed into her uterus like fancy fruit in a can. "So that's why she fought so hard," he thought. "It wasn't so much for her own life, it was the instinct to save her young. And we chased her and filled her full of green soap!"

"Doctors," he cried in the cold, white-filed aloneness of the autopsy room, "God-damn doctors!"

Then, quickly stripping off the gloves and gown and not even stopping to clean up, he fled the room and ran down the corridor. He felt sick and hoped he could make it to the bathroom in time.

Let Us All Pray

It was after dark when he arrived at the Pacific Garden Mission on skid row. The soup line had begun to queue up under the neon glare of the "Jesus Saves" sign, where both words used Jesus' middle 'S' in the center of the blinking cross. His friends of the Student Missionary Medical Fellowship assured him that his Jewishness would make no difference. Student physician volunteers were needed, and his services would be appreciated. But, as he approached the mission, he began to feel a little out of place.

Entering the lobby, with its worn, wine-colored carpet and plastic potted plants , he was suddenly confronted by a young Salvation Army lady in full regalia including cap and baton. "Major Barbara?" he asked, realizing immediately that the remark went well over her head and he should not anyway be so smart-mouthed. "No," she gently replied, "Lieutenant Sissons.

Can I assist you?" She directed him to where his group was meeting.

"Hi, Irv, glad you could make it." It was Chris Pearson, one of the Missionary Medical Fellows. Chris and four other medical students were lounging in the dispensary, the chips on the white-painted iron furniture catching the glare of an unshaded bulb hanging above them. The pungent smell of phenol bit at his nostrils. Introductions all around, and then they were oriented by a volunteer Christian Society senior physician.

"Now fellows, the important thing is not only to inquire into the physical complaint of the patient, but also to ask whether or not he has accepted Christ as his personal savior. Now then, the history, examination and treatment go on this side of the card." He demonstrated a plain 4 x 6 inch index card, "and whether or not he has accepted Christ as his personal savior and what he intends to do about it if he hasn't, go on the other side. It's best to clear up the religious convictions first, so that you can encourage the patient to save his soul, making it a part of the healing process. After the visit, you can give him a soup ticket, but tell him to attend the prayer meeting at 8 o'clock where the ticket will be stamped for the soup. Don't forget now, 'no prayer meeting, no stamp; no stamp, no soup.' Finally, you better let me see anyone who hasn't as yet accepted Christ as his personal savior. By the way, I'm also available should any medical problems come up. Questions?"

No questions, and they were off to the clinic.

The usual complaints for the mission. Lice, Scabies, two cases of DTs, all the backwash of poverty, filth and exposure. Dirty beards, rotten teeth, reddened eyes, black fingernails, torn jackets held together with safety pins and strings.

He had looked forward to playing doctor, and he was disappointed. They didn't need him. They didn't want help — not what he had to offer anyway. All they wanted was that bowl of soup and a warm bed for the night. And, if they could wangle it, a quarter for tomorrow's first drink. Several even tried to panhandle him out of that quarter. They all eagerly accepted, without question, Christ as their personal savior. They would have accepted Porky Pig or Allistair Cook, in fact, anyone or anything, upon which the soup and flop depended.

All over by 10 — then back to the dispensary for a report and windup.

"Good work, fellows," it was Doctor 'Personal Savior' again. "Not one religious holdout tonight. A perfect record. Let's celebrate it with a little prayer ring ourselves."

He gulped hard, but he was in too deep to back out. They sat in a ring in the middle of the clinic, joined hands and closed their eyes, each one reciting a prayer as they went around the circle counterclockwise. Fortunately, it started with Chris to his right, which gave him a few minutes to figure out his next move.

"Oh, Jesus," Chris began, "you have given me the strength to heal and the desire to help my fellow man. Oh, Christ my Lord and Savior ..." and on and on, through the next in line, and the man after him. Everyone sounded very experienced at the praying. Obviously, it was not the first time they had done this sort of thing. When it got to the man directly to his left, he figured that short of running for his life or disappearing into thin air, he had three viable alternatives. Either confess the fact that he was a non-Christian — this would embarrass him after his participation in the evening's activities; fake it — he was certain to feel guilty with this choice; or repeat the only prayers he knew by heart — these were the Hebrew Torah blessings from his Bar Mitzvah. The fourth alternative came to him just as his turn came up and the others looked toward him in quiet anticipation.

"Let us pray in silence," he said. And he smiled benignly as they all sighed and quietly lowered their heads.

Salvation

It happened while he was a junior medical student. He was assigned to the Chicago Maternity Center, delivering babies in ghetto apartments.

It was a cold night and there was no heat in the filthy two-room flat. It was the most depressing, seediest place he had ever been. Not a single piece of furniture was intact. The apartment was totally disordered. Three urchins, looking as if they had come directly from an anti-child-labor ad, were fending for themselves, and 3,000 roaches were having a holiday. The mother matched the environment, her haggard, strung-out look belying her given age of 25. It was a premature delivery in the eighth month of pregnancy. The fetus was not viable which seemed not to disappoint the father who sulked in the shadows. The mother was Catholic and a priest was called.

He was, hands down, the cleanest thing in the room; neatly dressed in his black suit and starched white clerical collar, clean-shaven, gentle touching and soft-spoken. He asked the exact moment of the death of the newborn. This was important because there was a strictly defined period during which salvation could be solicited for the unborn child. He breathed a sign of relief when he found he still had time to save the infant's soul. He placed the bloodied fetus, now wrapped in a newspaper, on the kitchen table, opening his satchel to remove the holy vestments, so he could begin his important task without delay.

In the meantime, the urchins fended for themselves, the roaches continued their holiday, the father sulked, and the mother quietly sobbed.

Poor No More

At that time, the medical internship was regarded as a privilege for which one was paid a pittance, if anything at all. His salary was $15 a month. He did not really mind it, though; the opportunity to put his newly acquired skills to work after four years of premed and another four of medical school was pay enough. Even anticipating another four years of residency training, the end was now in sight, and he knew they would make it, even with the child.

Toward the end of the year, he was notified that he had passed his state board examination and was licensed to practice medicine. A week after this, a friend of his asked him if he would like to sign on for emergency evening call through a local doctors' service.

"I never considered moonlighting. It's strictly against the rules, you know."

"That's true, but it's good experience, and I know you can use the money."

For a few days he wrestled with the moral dilemma of breaking the moonlighting rule of the hospital. If he was caught, there could be disciplinary action, even dismissal. He finally decided to do it. He told himself it was mostly for the experience, not the money.

The first call came during dinner. He could hardly suppress his excitement. He hastily put on a clean shirt and tie, checked his medical bag to make sure he had all his instruments, kissed his wife goodbye, assuring her he would return within the hour, and headed for his car.

Switching on the headlights of the car and pulling out into traffic, it suddenly occurred to him that for the first time he was treating a patient alone and he, and only he, would be fully responsible. He had never before felt such exhilaration. He suddenly realized that he was finally a physician.

Fortunately, the case was a simple one, a child with an upper respiratory tract infection. He spent almost an hour at the bedside, doing a much more thorough physical examination than required. He gave the necessary advice and prescribed the needed medications. The parents' deference was a feast for his ego. He felt 12 feet tall.

"How much do I owe you for the visit, Doctor?"

He didn't know what to respond.

"Well ... Five dollars ought to do it."

He didn't know it, but this was less than a third of the usual fee for a night call.

"Well, thank you much, Doctor. We certainly appreciate your coming out this time of night, and we are also thankful for your generosity."

"That's all right, Mrs. Grant, and don't worry about Nancy. She'll be just fine."

He checked with the service and found he had three more calls. After these he had two others. He traveled so much that evening, he had to find an all-night service station to get a refill of gasoline. All in all he had 21 house calls. He finally finished at 3:30 A.M.

He drove back to their small apartment through the now empty streets. His mind was supersaturated with the adventure of the evening, the challenge of each patient, the exercise of his diagnostic and therapeutic skills. Every house he passed was sleeping, but he felt wide awake. There was a hint of sunrise in the distance, and he was the only doctor in the world.

He softly let himself in, quietly entering the warmth of the apartment, putting down his medical bag, and removing his shoes at the front door, tiptoed carefully to the bedroom where his wife lay deep in sleep, their child in the crib beside her. He sat on the edge of the bed and looked at her for a few moments. Then gently touching her shoulder he whispered, "Darling, wake up, I've got something to show you." She stirred in her sleep, only slowly opening her eyes.

"Where have you been?" she whispered. "I was worried."

"Look what I have for you; we'll never be poor again."

With this he stood at the bedside, and reaching into every pocket he had, pulled out handfuls of one dollar bills. These he threw in the air over the bed onto which they settled like a layer of green dust in the early morning silence. There was more than $100.

"Poor no more, do you hear darling, poor no more!"

Poor no more, indeed, and it had nothing to do with the money. For that night he had validated his strength. It was the first time and the last, because he never felt so rich, in that special way, ever again.

THE ART

※ ※ ※

The great humanist/physician, Sir William Osler, observed that "The practice of medicine is an art based on science." Intellect isn't always the answer. As a doctor matures, intuition becomes more and more an active partner in his work.

"He has a nose for diagnosis, he seems to sense what's going on," we say of the experienced practitioner. And the use of this metaphor is no mere coincidence as smell is the most atavistic, intuitive sense we own. A physician must learn to trust intuition. If he is conscientious in his continuing education, he has probably learned many times over everything he needs to know in order to satisfy the demands of logic. The difficult task now is to search for where these facts converge. This does not involve more learning. It may even involve unlearning. If pursued, however, it ultimately brings him beyond the facts, even beyond knowledge, to wisdom. But careful, "Mother Nature" will, as often as not, tell you a direct lie if she can get away with it. What things are, are not always what they mean. Intuition, ah, intuition!

▨

What Do I Say?

The appointment was made in her name, and she had enough complaints for three visits and four doctors. He came along in tow.

"I just don't know where to start, Doctor. First, there's this feeling of being tired all the time. Then, every joint in my body aches, but the left shoulder and the right knee ..."

She hardly started to list her pains, when he interrupted, "She thinks she's got it bad. I'm so stiff in the morning I can hardly get out of bed to fetch aspirin for both of us," to which she replied:

"Aspirin won't touch the pain, Doctor. I really need something stronger. It must be something serious if aspirin won't touch it."

"Well, it doesn't help me either. I had to take two days off work last week, just because I couldn't sit for more than ten minutes without having terrific spasms in my back," he interjected.

"We have two heating pads, but one doesn't work so well. Every evening we have to decide which of us is the worse off and deserves the good heating pad," she added.

By this time, fascinated by the symptom symbiosis of their separate sicknesses, I suggested they might consider checking into a double room at the hospital for a mutual evaluation. Much to my dismay they took me seriously.

"That's a good idea. But would they permit a man and wife to occupy a double room?" he responded.

"Of course not, silly," she replied. "The doctor was only teasing us, weren't you, Doctor."

"Well, I ... " I stammered.

"Anyway, it's my appointment today and I'm the one who's here for an examination. You'll just have to wait your turn. Won't he, Doctor?"

"Well, I ... "

"You're being selfish, as usual, Maude. Doctor won't mind taking a look at me today. It'll only take a few minutes. What do you say, Doc?"

What do I say? I say that there is nothing new under the sun, that water seeks its own level, that the heart works in diastole as well as in systole, that a sense of humor always helps, and finally I say ... I think it's time for lunch!

❈

Research

The special value of scientific research, to paraphrase Francis Bacon, is not in how it changes the world, but in what it makes of the scientist. I speak, of course, of research as a state of mind, an attitude more than an engagement. It is a physician's responsibility to treat mankind as well as man. And in the syntax of daily practice, the attitude which looks to each patient as a unique problem of diagnosis and treatment is the hinge between the laboratory and the bedside. This viewpoint increases the doctor's response-ability, opening the door to some interesting observations otherwise not revealed.

Research need not limit itself to large clinical series. Many a new disease was first and best described on the basis of one well-documented case. Also, it is not always necessary to proceed from formalized training in research technique. Einstein, you'll remember, failed his entrance examination to the polytechnic school.

It has been pointed out that there is not that much difference between scientific discovery (Aha!), artistic creation (Ah!), and even humor (Ha, Ha!). They all tend to take what is known and look at it from a new perspective, thus demonstrating the unknown. As Louis Pasteur once noted, "To be astonished at anything is the first movement of the mind towards discovery."

This is not to claim that knowledge isn't necessary; luck does favor the "prepared mind." But sometimes a "creative ignorance" serves the task better. Witness Banting's and Best's discovery of insulin; ignorant that their ideas had already been tested and discarded, they innocently proceeded to discover the cause and treatment of diabetes.

I digress, however, from my original thesis, which is that the dialectic of research refines those faculties which are most useful in clinical practice. Play of the imagination, search for the exception, which, literally, proves the rule, the discovery of the beauty, indeed the truth of unity in variety. These things enliven and invigorate not only the practice of medicine but its practitioner as well.

It is given to few to move the world. It is within the capacity of each to make a small but meaningful and unique contribution by moving himself. The word "experiment" does not refer exclusively to the traditional laboratory. It derives from the Latin "experiri" which means "to try." Each of us carries a unique laboratory between our ears. And try each doctor should.

Life Goes On

L ife goes on.
"I have to see you, Doctor, right away!"

"What seems to be the trouble?"

"I have this pain in my foot. I simply can't bear it. I must see you!"

"I'm due in surgery shortly and my office is already heavily booked this afternoon. Perhaps I could give you some advice for temporary relief and have my secretary make an early appointment for you later this week ..."

"No, Doctor, that won't do. I simply must see you today!"

"Well, if it's an emergency."

"Yes, it certainly is an emergency!"

"Tell me what happened. How did the pain start?"

"I don't know what happened. It just started. I've had it for over three weeks now."

"Did you say three weeks? If you've had it for three weeks, it doesn't sound like much of an emergency to me."

"Well, three weeks or three months, it's an emergency to me, Doctor. Can't you see me today?"

"All right, if you are that concerned, I'll see you this afternoon. If you come in around 12:30 P.M., I'll see you before my regularly scheduled patients."

"That's not a good time for me. Can't you make it later, say about 4:30?"

"Why can't you make it at 12:30?"

"I have an appointment at the beauty parlor at noon which I wouldn't want to break."

Life goes on.

"Hello, Doctor, I've had this pain in my back for over two weeks now, and it's beginning to go down my right leg."

"How did it start? Did you injure yourself in some way?"

"Exactly, I bent over to hit a low shot in racquetball. I doubled up with pain and haven't been comfortable since."

"Have you noticed anything else? How about numbness in the leg?"

"How did you know? My whole foot is numb on that side. I even have difficulty standing on it."

"I think you'd better come in right away. I'll meet you in the hospital emergency room in an hour."

"I can't come in, Doctor, I have an important business conference later this morning. Can't you help me over the phone?"

"Now look, it sounds to me as if you have a slipped disc, and I think it's important that you see me today. We'll probably have to hospitalize you for this."

"That's impossible, Doctor. I'm due in New York City tomorrow to close a deal I've been working on for the last month. I've been making it to work every day on aspirin and a pair of crutches we had left over from my son's last football injury. All I need is something stronger for pain and some advice on how to treat this at home. I simply can't afford to come to the hospital right now."

"It's easy enough to get you some pain medication, but from what you tell me, I really feel you should be seen."

"I can't do it, Doctor. I'd like to, but I can't. It's impossible right now. Just get me the pain medication. Let me know what to do and I'll get back to you as soon as I can."

Life goes on.

We All Have Aliases

He used an assumed name when he registered in the emergency room. He had brought his collection of classical records, and these he gave to me saying he had no further need of them and wanted me to have them now.

He was one of the few black physicians I really knew, and we had been friends continuously and in a growing sense from the start of that knowing to the present. He was also the only pathologist I knew very well. That, I suppose, was a small part of the attraction, there being a little of the unexpressed necrophile in each of us. But mostly it was because he was so different.

He was young, handsome, single, drove a sports car, and lived with a white woman in a Bohemian neighborhood. I was older, married with four children, and lived in a sixteen room, 100-year-old house in a very respectable suburb. He was always troubled. Oversensitive, angry. He wrote poetry and listened to esoteric classical music. There was an aura of romanticism about his life. The struggle to rise from the ghetto. The civil rights movement. His swinging life style. He had even suffered tuberculosis, a classically "romantic" disease. After he resigned from our staff (the circumstances of his leaving were vague and never fully understood by me), he drifted from job to job. The last I heard of him was when we had lunch about a year ago and he told me he was leaving medicine because of what it had become and because of what he was becoming because of it. He planned to rest and think, to write poetry, and to listen to esoteric classical music. I remember my response at the time.

"Man," I said, making little attempt to conceal my envy, "what I wouldn't give to take a year off. You're living my fantasy. If I could only spend a year in an apartment in Old Town, sleeping with a black woman, writing poetry, and listening to good music."

That was the last I heard from Jim until he was brought to the emergency room by ambulance. He had, for some time, been living in a cold-water slum walk-up with a derelict woman he had picked up in a local tavern. They both were mainlining hard drugs. He hadn't enough money left to buy food. He had lost 70 pounds and looked as if his remaining 100 weren't at all going to make it. His arms and legs were covered with deep festering needle ulcers. What was left of his hands and feet was bloated beyond recognition. You didn't have to see him; the smell told you where he was.

"We all have aliases," I reflected. "Which of us is honest enough to admit to his own?" He was destroying himself. And that part of me which was linked to him was dying with him. There were now two deaths for me to grieve.

Later, I played the records he gave me. There was Bartok, Hindemith, Vivaldi, Shostakovich, Handel ...

My Problem

He was a middle-aged, single, unemployed mechanical engineer, and he was driving me crazy.

"My problem began a year ago. I call that Phase I. That was when I had the backache. I tried everything. Went from doctor to doctor with no relief. Finally, after three months, the backache left, and I began to go into Phase II. That was my period of sciatica. Again, no relief from anything. Physical therapy, injections, oral medications, braces, nothing seemed to help. About that time I was seeing my sixth or seventh orthopedic surgeon.

Then I went into Phase III, where the sciatica left and all I had was this persistent numbness in my left foot. Now I'm out of a job, out of funds, and on Public Aid. I have a pharmacist friend who gave me some of this new arthritis medication. I thought it might help because a doctor once told me I had some arthritis in my back. I read the package insert very carefully and followed the instructions to the letter. I immediately developed all the side effects mentioned in the package insert. I have a list here of all my complaints, as well as a diary detailing the progress of my illness over the last ten days. I've run out of treatments, medications, and now I'm running out of doctors. You're my last hope. Can you help me?"

I seriously doubt that I can help him. However, I simply have to try. That is my problem.

And so we enter Phase IV.

How Various, How Different They Were

"... only on the fringes of consciousness and in the deeper backgrounds into which they fade is freedom obtainable."
Brewster Ghiselin
The Creative Process

How various, how different they were.
Each his own formula,
authentic and unique.
Laennec rolling paper cylinders,
Augenbruger thumping kegs of wine,

Ehrlich tinkering in his dyes.
Like children at important games,
responsive only to that which they were doing.
Searching for something larger
than their own lives.

How similar, how alike they were.
Catalyzed by the same urgent vision.
Servitus burning at the stake.
Semmelweis maddened by his secret.
Morton dying in his cell.
Longing for what they could not themselves know.
Using and used completely.
Prison-pent by their restless hope.

What then is the process?
Fancy, wisdom, ideal, or thought?
Lister patient with his skill.
Pinel restless in his zeal.
Harvey at court
Beaumont alone.

Somewhere the crossing of the conscious
at the unconscious.
Sometime the outrageous conceit.
Somewhat the reasoned observation.
Somehow the errant dream.

Organan Language

" The standard nomenclature of disease" is a thorough clas-
sification of all human pathological states. Hospital
record rooms use it to code patient charts for statistical analysis and retrieval. Within its tables one can find catalogued every
variation and combination of every disease, including "no di-
agnosis-no known treatment", listed euphemistically as Yoo-Yoo
disease. Most Yoo-Yoo's represent psychosomatic problems;
that is, assuming, and such assumption is not always valid,
that organicity has been carefully ruled out. But show me someone who knows where the psyche ends and the soma begins,
and I'll show you a wise man indeed.

"I can't stomach my mother-in-law," complains the patient
with intermittent nausea, but a normal barium study of his G.I.
tract.

"This office routine is a pain in the neck," grumbles the
secretary whose physician finds muscle spasm, but nothing
else after a complete laboratory and x-ray workup, including a
neurological consultation.

"I can't swallow that."

"Get off my back."

"It's too much to shoulder."

Hypochondriacal means literally "below the ribs," and perhaps, such patients do hit us in this most vulnerable spot. But
Yoo-Yoo disease is real enough and the doctor's responsibility
(response-ability, the ability to respond) is to heal patients,
not only cure disease. This, indeed, is the difference between
the art and the craft of medicine.

India

"The last trip we made back home to India, we took him with us."

He couldn't take his eyes off her facial mark.

"We thought as long as no one here could offer us any hope of a cure, we would try some of the native Indian treatments."

It was a large magenta dot, smack in the middle of her forehead.

"He's so wasted and getting weaker all the time. We hoped against hope that the folk medicine of India would bring him to health."

He wondered what the mark meant.

"First we tried Hatha yoga. Then Reki-Reki."

Her sari also fascinated him.

"There was a local country practitioner who guaranteed us that massaging his arms and legs with the oil from the fat of a lion would bring him strength. We tried this also."

Its colors were muted and it was very sheer. He wondered how she wrapped it so that it looked like a dress.

"A friend told us of the urine treatment. It had to be his first urine of the day. We would let it stand for a week and then, after seasoning with various herbs and spices, he would drink it."

Her skin was the color of well-creamed coffee. She wore no lipstick.

"He seems a little stronger to me. Doctor. What do you think?

Her voice perfumed the room with incense. Her breath smelled of curry ... and of mantras.

High Finance

As one wag put it, "When I got the bill for my operation, I knew why the surgeon was wearing a mask!" Whether or not they should put the surgical recovery room next to the cashier's office is a moot point. We pay more for services and technology these days, and there seems no end in sight for our ever spiraling medical inflation. I honestly don't know what a brand new hip or knee is worth. At least as much as a five-year-old used Chevy, I suspect. I'd do the work for nothing, I enjoy it so much. I just wish my butcher, my baker and the mechanic who repairs my used Chevy felt the same way. How much something costs and what it's really worth are relative matters at best, particularly in a society which spends more on cigarettes and cosmetics than it does on health care and cancer research. Money shouldn't compromise medicine. Any lawyer will tell you that and sue you to prove it. An apple a day used to keep the doctor away, now it's the threat of a malpractice suit.

Fereida

Fereida was not one of those who twisted her diamond ring around so that the jewel faced her palm, assuming that I would charge her more if I saw the diamond and less if only the band were visible. She wouldn't do that if she could, and besides, she couldn't because she didn't have a diamond ring. She was truly poor, in money that is; in everything else she was rich beyond belief.

"Dottore, if you wanna da pepper, you better get me better by nexta time," she teased.

"Fereida, I'm doing the best I can. It must be all that pasta you eat. Besides making you fat, it neutralizes the medicines I give you," I gibed.

"Now, Doc, you know Italiano man lika da chubby woman. How I'ma gonna get me another fellow taka care of me in my olda age? I'ma pretty lonesome since Luigi die." She was widowed eighteen years.

"You're sixty-four years old now, Fereida. When do you anticipate entering this old age you speak about?"

"That'sa da nexta year, Doc, that'sa always da nexta year. Now, let'sa talk about something importante. You lika da bread I baka last time?"

"'Like' is the understatement of the year, Fereida. It was a culinary marvel. Absolutely the most delicious bread I ever tasted."

"Then I baka some more for you. But first, I make da peppers and tomatoes. Next, I fixa da home-made ravioli. Then I make da special sausage. I'm a gonna filla you up, Doc. I'ma gonna make you fat lika me."

He never charged her for the visits, simply allowing her to pay with gifts of food. Acting, at first, out of deference to her poverty, he came to regard the arrangement as very special. Her cooking was exceptional and he felt that he was getting the better of the bargain. Besides, the exchange pleased him in a strange way. He liked the idea of people paying for what they need with what they make, particularly if what they give comes of love and a sense of pride. It was honest and it was comfortable. It was intimate. It was, no doubt, the way things once were and should perhaps again be.

More Organ Language

"I went to work for four hours. I hate to tell you, I walked out of there like a cripple. Oh, my aching back!"

A thirty-two-year-old divorcee is talking.

"I don't know what I'm going to do about this back of mine. It's on again, off again. Some days good. Some days bad. But I'm never entirely rid of the pain."

"Did the physical therapy help at all?"

"It helps while I'm taking it, perhaps for a few hours afterwards. But it's hardly worth the trip and the expense for such temporary relief."

"We may have to hospitalize you again and keep you in traction."

"But I'm always better when I'm lying in bed. It's when I move around that it hurts. And besides, with all those fancy tests, you didn't find anything. You finally said it was just a chronic back strain."

"That's true. But if you're having such discomfort, we have no alternative."

"I thought once I unloaded that backbreaking divorce proceeding I'd be better, but it just hasn't worked out."

"Such things take time to get settled. They're never pleasant."

"I can't even have any decent sex life now. Intercourse aggravates the pain."

"I think it would be best if we hospitalized you again."

"Eight years I had my back to the wall in that lousy marriage. After the divorce I thought everything would improve. Isn't there something you can do for the pain? I can't seem to ever get rid of the pain."

❖

Love's Mysteries

"Love's Mysteries in souls do grow,
But yet the body is his book ...

The clinic had exhausted him. The counselling, especially. He sometimes had to reach far inside himself for answers, and often they weren't there. He knew, however, that she would be waiting for him when he got home.

They undressed each other slowly and, as always, with much tenderness.

A father is speaking of his two sons, both suffering muscular dystrophy, weakened, wasted, wheelchair-confined at age 14 and 15.

"The thing I feel worst about, well, you see, my wife and I have had a good marriage and we continue to love each other. Now I realize our sons will never walk again, nor even live much longer. But the thing I feel worst about is that they will never know the touch of a woman, that they will never experience the warmth of love."

He caressed her skin, waiting for the excitement to build and anticipating the sudden tightness in his groin. Yet all he felt was an odd and wonderful sense of enveloping warmth, of comfort, of peace.

A 21-year-old woman, handicapped by multiple sclerosis, is speaking.

"In spite of the fact that I want an intimate relationship so very much, I always hesitate at the idea. How may my mate see me as a handicapped person? Does he realize that there are points at which I could not go any further? How could I tell him how I feel at certain intimate moments? Could he sense my apprehension that he will notice the permanent catheter which drains my bladder? And suppose feeling has been lost in some parts of my body. How afraid I am that the other person might notice my lack of sensitivity and response. I guess

I'd have to pay very careful attention to where he was putting his hands, so as to make myself react as if I did feel him."

She began to stroke his body. First his face, then his back, his chest and abdomen, his thighs, his buttocks. Finally she gently curled the fingers of her right hand about his now stiffening organ while her left fondled the nape of his neck. Her warm tongue searched his mouth.

"My husband is so badly disfigured that intercourse is only possible if I shut my eyes or if it is absolutely dark." A young wife is speaking. "Then I can fantasize, more or less, that everything is just as it used to be."

He cupped the perfect white globes of her breasts. Her nipples swelled to the tender violence of his lips. How warm and moist she was where the sweet flesh parted between her smooth thighs. His fingers eagerly explored her openings.

John is 22 years old and suffers from a severe spastic condition. He is of above normal mentality and is studying psychology at the university level. He lives at home with his parents. He is wheelchair-confined.

"It is easier discussing things with men, especially with young fellows, and if they start talking about their sexual experiences, I can really appreciate it. This usually means that they regard me as a man, not a disabled creature. However, personal contacts are harder to make with girls. I find it impossible to ask someone, 'Let's make love together,' because when I look at myself in the mirror, the deformed figure is horrifying, and I can understand how others might be similarly appalled."

Now, yes, yes, oh yes, now they were eagerly upon each other. His open mouth between her open legs her lips tightening about his swelling sex.

A woman of 34, severely crippled by rheumatoid arthritis.

"I should like to use a vibrator for masturbating, but because of my deformities, I cannot hold such a thing and reach my genitals. Special spoon and fork holders have been designed to aid rehabilitation. Has something similar been done with a vibrator?"

169

How gently and modestly she fits herself to him, measuring and meeting his need. He surrenders fully to the wonder of her readiness. Now mounting and urgently entering her body.

An uncle inquiring about his disabled nephew. "As you know, Doctor, he's 24 and bed-bound. He can't even turn or clean himself. He knows he's going to die soon and he asked me to bring him a woman. I'd be glad to do it, but his mother thinks it's sinful and she'll hear nothing of it. What do you think, Doctor? Is it wicked? Is it wrong? Will you talk to her for me?"

She opens like a hungry flower. He thrust deep and again into her warm corridor until finally he found himself. She gasped as their love glands burst.

"Even though I am 26, I have never attempted to make love to a woman." He stares into nothingness as he talks. "When you are blind, like I am, you never know how you are being accepted, nor do you know just how to act. I don't even know what a woman looks like. This is very sad to me. It's not as if I were just missing an experience. It's more like I was missing a part of myself."

To our bodies turn we then, that weak men on love revealed may look; Love's mysteries in souls do grow, but yet the body is his book..."

John Donne
"The Ecstasy"

❖

The Dream Fish

"Of a truth, men are mystically united, a mysterious bond of brotherhood makes all men one."
                                                    Carlyle

*"It is generally believed today that life began
                                    in the sea..."*
                                        Baldwin
                        Comparative Biochemistry

The heart hangs from its aorta
Like a ripe plum.

Tight in the joy and the pain
Of its rhythm.
As it beats, does the sea still move
Within us,

Sweeping the shores
Of a distant consciousness?

The blood should remember
What the brain is too young to know.

The sound of magic thunder,
The smell of the rock,
The taste of earth.

For deep beneath the sea
I feel
The dream fish move.

Their lungs thick
With the lymph
Of an inarticulate desire.

Their secret, silent voices whispering
Down my veins.

Celebrating the joy and pain of man.
Sharing the sun-warmth of a single skin,
Breathing the sea tide of a common blood.

EPILOGUE

⊠⊠⊠

I remember something here. What is it?

Is it the music they pipe into the clinic so you can examine the spastics and the amputees to the gentle background strains of "Love is a Many Splendored Thing," played by Andre Kastelanitz and his singing violins?

Is it the fact that men have been known to ejaculate at the very moment of violent death?

Or is it the restraints the nurses' aides used to tie down elderly patients on Ward 15 at County Hospital so they couldn't wander about at night when they became confused by the dark? I remember that some of these were cardiacs who couldn't sleep lying flat, and they would gasp for breath as they tried unsuccessfully to sit up in bed. The restraints were made of leather.

Perhaps it is the leper colony I remember, with the iron gate and its ancient bell tolled by a frayed rope knotted at the end. There was enough pain behind that gate to twice fill any lifetime.

Maybe I recall what is written on the gravestone of the great surgeon, Nicholas Senn, buried in the Graceland Cemetery of Chicago: "Nihil sans labore," it says, "nothing without labor."

Or perhaps I have simply been too long in a place with too many people whose first name is "Doctor"?

A condition of the mind, you say, something I should forget? Should I then forget all those ill and all the diseases, even those recognized in strangers, in passersby, even the skin cancer diagnosed at a glance on the face of the man sitting next to me on the bus?

Yes, all of it is stored neatly in the computer, ready for instant replay.

I remember something here. What is it?

Is it the lady who on admission to the hospital requested a bed in which no one had ever died? Or the one who wrote me a letter asking how her "testes" had come out?

Is it Room 101 in Orwell's novel, *1984,* which held the worst thing in the world? This thing was different for everyone and each had to make his own choice. The room, by the way, was under the authority of the Minister of Love.

I remember other rooms; I remember the "serious rooms" at the charity hospital where they put the dying patients most likely to succeed, and the patients knew it. "Go to the morgue," the doctor said. "Go directly to the morgue. Do not pass the pharmacy. Do not stop at surgery. Do not collect a cure."

What do I remember? My first delivery, perhaps. And sitting on the dark fire escape afterwards, alone and weeping without shame at the pain and the wonder of the infinite mystery of the only miracle there is.

I remember something here. Half in flight and half in pursuit, I pause to recollect. Memories which reach from hope to despair, from grief to celebration. More than an act of witness I remember, rather an act of involvement.

What it has been;

what it is;

what it can become.